PROSTATE CANCER

A PRACTICAL GUIDE

May Abdel-Wahab MD, PhD
Associate Professor of Radiation Oncology & Residency Program Director,
Department of Radiation Oncology, Sylvester Comprehensive Cancer Center,
University of Miami Miller School of Medicine, Florida, USA

Orlando E. Silva MD, JD, FACP, FCLM
Associate Professor of Medicine, Sylvester Comprehensive Cancer Center,
University of Miami Miller School of Medicine, Florida, USA

SAUNDERS

ELSEVIER

EDINBURGH LONDON NEW YORK OXFORD PHILADELPHIA
ST LOUIS SYDNEY TORONTO 2008

SAUNDERS
ELSEVIER

First published 2008

ISBN: 978-0-7020-2890-8

British Library Cataloguing in Publication Data
A catalogue record for this book is available from the British Library

Library of Congress Cataloging in Publication Data
A catalog record for this book is available from the Library of Congress

Notice
Knowledge and best practice in this field are constantly changing. As new research and experience broaden our knowledge, changes in practice, treatment and drug therapy may become necessary or appropriate. Readers are advised to check the most current information provided (i) on procedures featured or (ii) by the manufacturer of each product to be administered, to verify the recommended dose or formula, the method and duration of administration, and contraindications. It is the responsibility of the practitioner, relying on their own experience and knowledge of the patient, to make diagnoses, to determine dosages and the best treatment for each individual patient, and to take all appropriate safety precautions. To the fullest extent of the law, neither the Publisher nor the Editors assumes any liability for any injury and/or damage to persons or property arising out or related to any use of the material contained in this book.   *The Publisher*

Working together to grow libraries in developing countries

www.elsevier.com | www.bookaid.org | www.sabre.org

ELSEVIER   **BOOK AID International**   Sabre Foundation

ELSEVIER   your source for books, journals and multimedia in the health sciences
www.elsevierhealth.com

The publisher's policy is to use paper manufactured from sustainable forests

Printed in China.

PROSTATE
CANCER

Dedication

This book is dedicated to our past and future patients who taught us through their courage and perseverance; to our residents and fellows for their inquisitiveness and their questions; to our mentors past and present, in particular the late Professor Dr Hassan Awad.

Most importantly, this is dedicated to our parents for their support, patience and guidance, and spouses, and children, Nora and Ahmed, for inspiring us to make a difference.

For Elsevier

Commissioning Editor: Pauline Graham
Development Editor: Barbara Simmons
Project Manager: Susan Stuart
Typesetting and Production: Helius
Illustrations: Barking Dog
Designer: George Ajayi

Acknowledgments

The editors would like to thank the following contributing experts for actively participating and offering invaluable advice in the preparation of this handbook. Some helped with the entirety of the book and some with specific chapters as listed under their names.

May Abdel-Wahab MD, PhD
(Chapters 12, 16)
Associate Professor of Radiation Oncology,
Department of Radiation Oncology,
University of Miami Miller School of Medicine,
Miami, Florida, USA

Abdullah Sakher MD
(Chapter 1)
Hematology and Oncology Fellow,
Department of Medicine,
Division of Medical Oncology,
University of Miami Miller School of Medicine,
Miami, Florida, USA

Robin Scott Akins MD
(Chapter 9)
Resident,
Department of Radiation Oncology,
University of Miami Miller School of Medicine,
Miami, Florida, USA

Marco Amendola MD
(Chapter 6)
Professor of Radiology,
Department of Radiology,
University of Miami Miller School of Medicine,
Miami, Florida, USA

Rajinikanth Ayyathurai MD, MS, MRCS(Ed)
(Chapter 5)
Senior Research Associate –
Urology,
University of Miami Miller School of Medicine,
Miami, Florida, USA

K. C. Balaji MD, FRCS
(Chapters 17, 24)
Professor and Chairman,
Department of Urology,
University of Massachusetts,
Worchester, Massachusetts, USA

Matt Biagioli MD, MSc
(Chapters 14, 25)
Chief Resident,
Department of Radiation Oncology,
University of Miami Miller School of Medicine,
Miami, Florida, USA

Marcello Blaya MD
(Chapter 18)
Hematology and Oncology Fellow,

Department of Medicine,
Division of Medical Oncology,
University of Miami Miller School
of Medicine,
Miami, Florida, USA

Inas Elattar DMD, DrPH
(Chapter 2)
Professor and Chair,
Department of Biostatistics and
Cancer Epidemiology,
National Cancer Institute,
Cairo University,
Cairo, Egypt

Nagy Elsayyad MD
(Chapter 19)
Assistant Professor,
Harvard University Medical
School,
Boston, Massachusetts, USA

D. Scott Ernst MD
(Chapters 4, 18, 19, 20, 21, 22, 23)
Associate Professor of Medicine,
Department of Medicine,
Division of Medical Oncology,
University of Miami Miller School
of Medicine,
Miami, Florida, USA

Hyo Han MD
(Chapter 4)
Hematology and Oncology Fellow,
Department of Medicine,
Division of Medical Oncology,
University of Miami Miller School
of Medicine,
Miami, Florida, USA

Alejandra Izaguirre MD
(Chapter 13)
Fellow,
Department of Radiation Oncology,
University of California in San
Francisco (UCSF),
San Francisco, California, USA

Merce Jorda MD, PhD
(Chapter 8)
Associate Professor of Pathology,
Department of Pathology,
University of Miami Miller School
of Medicine,
Miami, Florida, USA

Bruce Kava MD
(Chapters 7, 15)
Assistant Professor of Urology,
University of Miami Miller School
of Medicine,
Miami, Florida, USA

Prasanna Kumar MD
(Chapter 6)
Radiologist,
Roswell Park Cancer Institute,
Buffalo, New York, USA

Christopher Lobo MD
(Chapters 10, 19)
Hematology and Oncology Fellow,
Department of Medicine,
Division of Medical Oncology,
University of Miami Miller
School of Medicine,
Miami, Florida, USA

Gilberto Lopes MD
(Chapter 22)
Hematology and Oncology Fellow,
Department of Medicine,
Division of Medical Oncology,
University of Miami Miller School
of Medicine,
Miami, Florida, USA

Tony Mammen MD
(Chapters 17, 24)
Resident in Urology,
University of Nebraska Medical
Center,
Omaha, Nebraska, USA

Murugesan Manoharan MD
(Chapters 5, 11, 15, 26)
Associate Professor of Urology,

University of Miami Miller School
of Medicine,
Miami, Florida, USA

David Meinbach MD
(Chapter 26)
Chief Resident in Urology,
University of Miami School of
Medicine,
Miami, Florida, USA

Subhakar Mutyala MD
(Chapter 14)
Assistant Professor and Director
of Brachytherapy Service,
Montefiore Medical Center,
Albert Einstein College of
Medicine of Yeshiva University,
New York, USA

Alan M. Nieder MD
(Chapters 11, 15)
Assistant Professor of Urology,
University of Miami Miller School
of Medicine,
Miami, Florida, USA

Janet Nguyen MD
(Chapter 18)
Resident,
Department of Radiation Oncology,
University of Miami Miller School
of Medicine,
Miami, Florida, USA

Mack Roach III MD
(Chapter 13)
Professor and Chairman,
Department of Radiation
Oncology,
University of California in San
Francisco (UCSF),
San Francisco, California, USA

Eloy Roman MD
(Chapter 21)
Hematology and Oncology Fellow,
Department of Medicine,
Division of Medical Oncology,

University of Miami Miller School
of Medicine,
Miami, Florida, USA

Manuel Rosado MD
(Chapter 10)
Assistant Professor of Oncology,
Yale University,
New Haven, Connecticut, USA

Alvaro Saenz MD
(Chapter 8)
Resident,
Department of Pathology,
University of Miami Miller School
of Medicine,
Miami, Florida, USA

Shalin Shah MD
(Chapter 14)
Resident,
Department of Radiation Oncology,
Montefiore Medical Center,
Albert Einstein College of
Medicine of Yeshiva University,
New York, USA

Orlando E. Silva MD, JD, FACP, FCLM
(Chapter 21)
Associate Professor of Medicine,
University of Miami Miller School
of Medicine,
Miami, Florida, USA

Rakesh Singal MD
(Chapters 4, 20, 23)
Associate Professor of Medicine,
Department of Medicine,
Division of Medical Oncology,
University of Miami Miller School
of Medicine,
Miami, Florida, USA

Mark Soloway MD
(Chapter 15)
Professor and Chair,
Department of Urology,
University of Miami, Miller School
of Medicine,
Miami, Florida, USA

Alexandra Stefanovic MD
(Chapters 2, 23)
Hematology and Oncology Fellow,
Department of Medicine,
Division of Medical Oncology,
University of Miami Miller School
of Medicine,
Miami, Florida, USA

Samuel P. Sterrett MD
(Chapters 17, 24)
Resident in Urology,
University of Nebraska Medical
Center,
Omaha, Nebraska, USA

Michel Vulfovich MD
(Chapter 3)
Hematology and Oncology Fellow,
Department of Medicine,
Division of Medical Oncology,
University of Miami Miller School
of Medicine,
Miami, Florida, USA

Eric Winquist MD
(Chapter 23)
Associate Professor of Medicine,
University of Western Ontario,
London, Ontario, Canada

How to use this book

This handbook is written to be a 'bedside' reference for radiation oncologists and medical oncologists, as well as a compendium of prostate cancer information useful to urologists, clinical researchers and educators, medical students, and nurses.

The book is written telegraphically, in outline format, emphasizing the key concepts. By this means, the reader has an immediately accessible portal to the current literature, the major trials, the landmark articles, and the reviews. The results of important trials are summarized in 5–10 lines, with key data including: whether or not randomized, number of subjects, study period, median follow-up, dosages, results, limitations, and conclusions. In addition, there is a comprehensive index so that specific information can be found quickly.

It is our hope that this compendium will not only be an aid to the physician in patient care, but also to the physician scientists, as it indicates where knowledge is lacking and understanding is incomplete, suggesting targets for future research. We plan to continue publishing periodic updates as progress in combating this major health problem continues.

Commonly used abbreviations

A2M	α-2-Macroglobulin	CI	Confidence interval
ACT	α-1-Antichymotrypsin	CLL	Chronic lymphatic leukemia
AAPM	American Association of Physicists in Medicine	cPSA	Complexed prostate-specific antigen
AD	Androgen deprivation	CT	Computerized tomography
ADT	Androgen-deprivation therapy	3D	Three-dimensional
AMACR	α-Methylacyl-coenztme A racemase	3D-CT	Three-dimensional conformal therapy
AP	Anteroposterior	DBCG 82c	Danish Breast Cancer Cooperative Group 82c
API	α-1-Trypsin inhibitor	DFS	Disease-free survival
AR	Androgen receptor	DHT	Dihydrotestosterone
ASAP	Atypical small acinar proliferation	DRE	Digital rectal examination
ASCO	American Society of Clinical Oncology	EBRT	External beam radiation therapy
ASTRO	American Society for Therapeutic Radiology and Oncology	ECE	Extracapsular extension
		ECOG	Eastern Cooperative Oncology Group
ATBC	Alpha-Tocopherol, Beta Carotene Cancer Prevention [Trial]	ELND	Extended lymph node dissection
AUA	American Urological Association	EORTC	European Organisation for Research and Treatment of Cancer
b.i.d	Twice daily	fPSA	Free prostate-specific antigen
BMP	Bone morphogenetic protein	GM-CSF	Granulocyte-macrophage colony-stimulating factor
BPH	Benign prostatic hyperplasia	GSTP1	Glutathione S-transferase gene
bRFS	Biochemical relapse-free survival	HBI	Hemibody irradiation
CAB	Combined androgen blockade	HDR	High dose rate
		HGP	Human Genome Project
CALGB	Cancer and Leukemia Group B	HGPIN	High-grade prostatic intraepithelial neoplasia
CaPSURE	Cancer of the Prostate Strategic Urologic Research Endeavor	hK2	Human kallikrein 2
		HMWK	High molecular weight cytokeratin
CARET	Beta-Carotene and Retinol Efficacy [Trial]	HR	Hazard ratio

HRPC	Hormone-refractory prostate cancer	PFS	Progression-free survival
HRQOL	Health-related quality of life	PIN	Prostatic intraepithelial neoplasia
IAS	Intermittent androgen suppression	PLN	Pelvic lymph node
ICRU	International Committee on Radiation Units and Measurements	PLND	Pelvic lymph node dissection
		PNET	Primitive peripheral neuroectodermal tumor
		p.o.	By mouth
IGF	Insulin-like growth factor	PR	Partial response
IGFBP	Insulin-like growth factor binding protein	PR	Progesterone receptor
		PSA	Prostate-specific antigen
IGFR	Insulin-like growth factor receptor	PSADT	Prostate-specific antigen doubling time
i.m.	Intramuscular	PSMA	Prostate-specific membrane antigen
IMRT	Intensity-modulated radiation therapy	PTEN	Phosphatase and tensin homologue
IU	International units		
i.v.	Intravenous	PTV	Planning target volume
LDR	Low dose rate	q	Every
LFTs	Liver function tests	QOL	Quality of life
LH	Luteinizing hormone	Rb	Retinoblastoma
LHRH	Luteinizing hormone releasing hormone	RFS	Relapse-free survival
		RR	Relative risk
LN	Lymph node	RRP	Radical retropubic prostatectomy
LT LAT	Left lateral		
ml	Milliliter	RT	Radiotherapy
MRI	Magnetic resonance imaging	RT LAT	Right lateral
MRS	Magnetic resonance spectroscopy	RTOG	Radiation Therapy Oncology Group
NBS1 gene	Nijmegen Breakage Syndrome	RT-PCR	Reverse transcription polymerase chain reaction
NCI	National Cancer Institute		
NCIC	National Cancer Institute of Canada	s.c.	Subcutaneous
		SEER	Surveillance, Epidemiology, and End Results
ng	Nanogram		
NIST	National Institutes of Standards and Technology	SELECT	Selenium and Vitamin E Cancer Prevention [Trial]
NLCS	Netherlands Cohort Study	SLL	Small lymphocytic lymphoma
NSAID	Non-steroidal anti-inflammatory drug	SLN	Sentinel lymph node
		SPECT	Single photon emission computerized tomography
OS	Overall survival		
PA	Posteroanterior	SRE	Skeletal-related event
PAP	Prostatic alkaline phosphatase	SU.VI.MAX	Supplementation of Vitamins and Mineral Antioxidants [Trial]
PCPT	Prostate Cancer Prevention Trial		
		SVI	Seminal vesicle invasion
PCR	Polymerase chain reaction	SWOG	Southwest Oncology Group
PDE-5	Phosphodiesterase type-5	TGF-β1	Transforming growth factor-β1
PDGF	Platelet-derived growth factor	TGF-β2	Transforming growth factor-β2
PEComa	Perivascular epithelioid cell tumor	t.i.d.	Three times daily
		tPSA	Total prostate-specific antigen

TRT	Testosterone-replacement therapy	VDR	Vitamin D receptor
TRUS	Transrectal ultrasonography	VEGF	Vascular endothelial growth factor
TURP	Transurethral resection of the prostate	vs	Versus, or compared to
VACURG	Veterans Administration Cooperative Urological Research Group	WPRT	Whole-pelvic radiotherapy
		♀	Woman or female
		♂	Man or male

Contents

Contents

History of prostate cancer

- 2650 BC: Imhotep, an Egyptian physician, architect, and astrologer during the third dynasty, who also designed the first pyramid at Saqqara and was called the god of healing.
  - During that time early Egyptians documented breast cancer and treated the tumors by cautery of the diseased tissue.

- 1700 BC: the code of Hammurabi was commissioned in Babylon; it provided the first written laws that regulated, among other things, the responsibilities and fees of medical practitioners and physicians.

- 1700 BC: An Egyptian medical treatise was written that contained descriptions of surgical procedures, examination, diagnosis, treatment, prognosis, and drugs, in addition to anatomy.
  - It was later acquired by Edwin Smith and presented to the New York Historical Society in 1906.

- One of the oldest available specimens of a human cancer was found in the remains of the skull of a female who lived during the Bronze Age (1900–1600 BC).
  - The tumor in the women's skull was suggestive of head and neck cancer.
  - The mummified skeletal remains of Peruvian Incas, dating back 2400 years ago, contained abnormalities suggestive of involvement with malignant melanoma.
  - Cancer was also found in fossilized bones recovered from ancient Egypt.

- Hippocrates, the great Greek physician (460–370 BC), who is

considered the father of medicine, is thought to be the first person to clearly recognize the difference between benign and malignant tumors.
- His writings include a description of cancers involving various body sites.

- Hippocrates noticed that blood vessels around a malignant tumor looked like the claws of crab. He named the disease *karkinos* (the Greek name for crab) to describe tumors that may or may not progress to ulceration. In English this term translates to 'carcinos' or 'carcinoma'.

- Works of Hippocrates and Galen, another Greek physician, revolutionized the practice of medicine by removing it from the grip of superstitions and magic, to the era of observation and logical reasoning.

- Later in the course of history, Constantinople became the intellectual headquarters of medicine.
  - The ancient teachings of Hippocrates and Galen continued to influence the physicians in Constantinople, Cairo, Alexandria, and Athens.
  - During this period the cause of cancer was explained to be an 'excess of black bile'.

- 865–923 AD: Al-Razi, born in Rayy (now in Iran) and wrote in Arabic. George Sarton said: 'Rhazes was the greatest physician of Islam and the Medieval Ages.' He is credited with the discovery of sulfuric acid, and ethanol and its refinement and use in medicine.
  - He wrote 184 books and articles in various fields of science. One of the most famous books is *Al-Hawi* (*The Continence*).
  - Razi was the first physician to diagnose smallpox and measles, and the first to distinguish the difference between them. He is also known for having discovered 'allergic asthma', and was the first physician ever to write an article on allergy and immunology.
  - He commented that in advanced cases of cancer and leprosy the physician should not be blamed when he could not cure them.
  - He said: 'Truth in medicine is an unattainable goal, and the art as described in books is far beneath the knowledge of an experienced and thoughtful physician.'

- 980–1037 AD: Avicenna (Ibn Sina), born in Afshana (now part of Uzbekistan). A Muslim physician, philosopher, and scientist of Persian-Tajik origin.
  - He wrote in Arabic and was the author of 450 books and articles on a wide range of subjects, mainly philosophy and medicine.
  - George Sarton called Ibn Sina 'the most famous scientist of Islam and one of the most famous of all races, places, and times.'

- His most famous works are *Kitab al-shifa* (*The Book of Healing*) and *al-Qanoun fil-Tib* (*The Rules of Medicine*), also known as the *Qanun*, which was a standard medical text in western Europe for seven centuries, after being translated into Latin by Gerard of Cremona.
- There is a crater on the moon called Avicenna, which is named after him.

- 1213–1288 AD: Ibn Al-Nafis, born in Damascus, Syria. He attended the Medical College Hospital (Bimaristan Al-Noori). Apart from medicine, Ibn al-Nafis learned jurisprudence, literature, and theology.
  - He was the first physician to disagree with Galen's teachings and to present the correct and currently accepted knowledge about the pulmonary circulation, the anatomy of the heart, and the coronary circulation.
  - In 1628 this discovery would be rediscovered, or perhaps merely demonstrated, by William Harvey, who generally receives the credit in western history.
  - Ibn Al-Nafis was only credited for what he did after the reading and translation of some of his writings, which were preserved in Germany by an Egyptian scholar in 1924.

- 1793 AD: Mathew Baille of St. George Hospital, London, published *Morbid Anatomy of Some of the Most Important Parts of the Human Body*.
  - It contained descriptions of the symptoms and morbid anatomy of cancer of the esophagus, stomach, bladder, and testis, and was generally regarded as reaching new heights of clarity in the history and classification of oncology.

- 1805–1884: Samuel David Gross, an American surgeon who introduced laparotomy for ruptured bladder, suprapubic incision for the prostate, distinguished prostatic hypertrophy from bladder disease, and wrote *Elements of Pathological Anatomy*.

- 1820: the first description of cancer due to arsenic was given by John Ayrton, a physician from Penzance, England.

- 1820: Sir Henry Thompson was born. He was an English surgeon who described the surgical treatment of urinary bladder tumors, and was one of the first surgeons who wrote extensively on prostate cancer.

- 1829: The term 'metastasis' to describe the spread of cancer was introduced by French gynecologist and obstetrician Joseph Recalmier.

- 1830: Everard Home, an English surgeon, was the first to illustrate the appearance of cancer cells under the microscope.

3

- 1836–1921: Heinrich Wilhelm Von Wladeyer-Hartz, a German histologist, classified the emergence of carcinomas from epithelial cells, and sarcoma from mesodermal tissue.

- 1837: John Collins Warren wrote the first American book on tumors, *Surgical Observations on Tumors with Cases and Operations.*

- 1845: Wilhelm Konrad Rontgen was born. He was a German physicist and Nobel Laureate (1901) who discovered x-rays in 1895.

- 1851: The distinction between carcinoma and hypertrophy of the prostate was made by the English surgeon John Adams.

- 1860: Jean Danysz was born. He was a Polish pathologist who applied radium to malignant tumors.

- 1861: William James Mayo was born. He was one of the great reformers of American medicine and a co-founder of the Mayo clinic.

- 1875: Henry Khunrath Pancoast was born. He was a Philadelphia radiologist and pioneer in the use of radiotherapy (Pancoast tumor, 1932).

- 1895: The discovery that certain substances, such as uranium salts, emitted radiation similar to x-rays was made by the French physicist Anotine Becquerel, and the phenomenon was later named 'radioactivity' by Pierre and Marie Curie, who later discovered and isolated the radioactive elements polonium and radium.

- 1901: Charels Brenton Huggins was born. He was a Canadian-born American surgeon who pioneered the hormonal treatment of cancer, investigated the physiology of the male urogenital tract, and developed a diagnostic test for cancer and an operation for prostate cancer. He died in 1997.

- 1905: George Hitchings was born. He was an American biochemist and Nobel Laureate (1988) who discovered the folic acid antagonist, 2-aminopurine (1948), the antimalarial agent pyrimethamine (1952), the antileukemia drug 6-mercaptopurine, and the immunosuppressant drugs azathioprine (1965) and zidovudine.

- 1907: The American Association for Cancer Research was established by a group of leading pathologists, including James Ewing.

- In 1913, a need to combat rising public fear and ignorance concerning cancer led to two significant events: the publication in a popular woman's magazine of the first known article on the warning signs of cancer, and the formation of a nationwide organization dedicated to public education about cancer. Cancer, as a disease, was brought into the light of day.

- 1920: Charles Heidelberger was born. He was a professor of oncology at Wisconsin, who introduced fluorouracil as a tumor-inhibiting compound.

- 1926: The German biochemist Otto Wargurg made the discovery that malignant cells use glucose by glycolysis, in the presence or absence of oxygen, a discovery that is well appreciated in the treatment modalities of cancer.

- 1937: The US Congress made the conquest of cancer a national goal, with a unanimous vote to pass the National Cancer Institute Act. This Act created the National Cancer Institute, which was expected to break new theoretical ground by conducting its own research, promoting research in other institutions, and coordinating cancer-related projects and activities.

- 1938: Benjamin Barringer and H Woodward, two New York surgeons, documented that metastatic prostate cancer causes elevation of serum levels of acid phosphatase.

- 1938: Temple Fay used cryotherapy for the treatment of carcinoma.

- 1939: Alfred Loeser and Paul Ulrich used testosterone in the treatment of prostate carcinoma.

- 1939: Radioactive isotopes were employed for the first time in the treatment of leukemia by John Lawrence and co-workers.

- 1941: A Canadian-born American urologist, Charles Huggins, noted that metastatic carcinoma of the prostate responded positively to treatment with estrogenic substances.

- The TNM (tumor, node, metastasis) classification for cancer was proposed by P. Denois of the Institute Gustav–Roussay in France.

- 1946: Frederick S. Phillips and Alfred Gilman made the discovery that nitrogen mustards could bring about regression of certain lymphomas and leukemias, a landmark development in cancer therapy.

- 1948: Methotrexate was developed from aminopterin by Sidney Farber, a cancer scientist in the USA, as a treatment for leukemia. It was later used to cure choriocarcinoma by Li and Hartz.

- 1948: The World Health Organisation was established by the United Nations.

- 1960: M. E. Hodes and colleagues used vincaleukoblastine (from Madagascar periwinkle) in the treatment of leukemia.
  - This later led to the development of vincristine.
- 1965: Barnett Rosenberg of Michigan State University discovered cisplatin, a dissolved form of platinum later shown by others to interfere with DNA prior to cell division.
  - Cisplatin is now one of the most used chemotherapeutic agents in the treatment of cancer.
- 1971: A cure for childhood cancer, acute lymphoblastic leukemia, was found by Donald Pinkel of St. Jude's Hospital, Memphis, USA. He used combined chemotherapy and radiation therapy.
- 1971: The National Cancer Act was launched, a National Cancer Program administered by the National Cancer Institute.
- 1973: Computerized axial tomography (CAT) was invented by Sir Godfrey Newbold Hounsfield and Allan Macleod Cormack, in Britain and America, independently.
- 1976: The Argentine immunologist Cesar Milstein and the German molecular biologist Georges Kohler created hybridomas by fusing cultured myeloma cells with normal B cells from the spleen of an immunized mouse.
- 1977: Cyproterone acetate was used in the treatment of prostatic carcinoma by D. Y. Wang and R. D. Bulbrook.
- 1978: The cancer suppressor *p53* gene was discovered by David Lane, a Professor of Oncology at Dundee, Scotland.
- History of prostate-specific antigen.
  - 1960s: Ablin and co-workers reported novel proteins found in seminal fluid.
  - 1971: In the *Japanese Journal of Legal Medicine*, Hara and co-workers identified what they considered a protein unique to semen. They were attempting to find a substance in seminal fluid that would aid in the investigation of rape cases.
  - 1973: Li and Beling isolated and purified this protein.
  - 1978: Sensabaugh characterized this protein as a semen-specific protein; he referred to it as p30 because of its molecular weight.
  - 1979: Perhaps the most important contribution in the development of this test was the report by Wang and co-workers at Roswell Park, Buffalo, NY. In 1979, they published a paper in *Investigative Urology* in which they described the isolation of a tissue-specific antigen

from the prostate using gel electrophoresis. They called this 'prostate-specific antigen' (PSA). Further study by Wang and co-workers demonstrated that this protein was immunologically identical to the one discovered by Hara and Sensabaugh.

- 1980: Papsidero, Wang and co-workers developed a serologic test allowing PSA to be measured in the serum.
- 1987: Stamey and co-workers at Stanford University published the first definitive clinical study investigating the utility of PSA in prostate cancer. Since then there has been extensive investigation into the various uses of this protein.

- The last 25 years: Different modes of therapy have been used in different stages of the disease: surgery, radiation therapy, and cryotherapy in localized, non-meastatic disease (radiation therapy for palliative goals also); androgen depletion strategies using orchiectomy; luteinizing hormone releasing hormone (LHRH) agonists, estrogens, and anti-androgens are also used at different stages of the disease.

- Renewed interest in the research of prostate cancer has emerged lately, and currently there are at least 250 studies recruiting in the USA, using different old and new treatment modalities, and including the new targeted agents that interfere with the growth pathways, signal transduction pathways, vascular endothelial growth factor (VEGF) pathway, and monoclonal antibodies.

- 2000: A rough draft of the human genome was finished in 2000 (announced jointly by US President Bill Clinton and British Prime Minister Tony Blair on June 26, 2000), 2 years earlier than planned. This work was done by the Human Genome Project (HGP) and was started in the early 1980s. In addition to workers in the USA, the international consortium comprised geneticists from China, France, Germany, Japan, and the UK.

- Eight years after the HGP was begun, an identical quest was initiated separately with private venture capital by a company called Celera Genomics (founded by Craig Venter), while the HGP was still being pursued.
  - Celera Genomics used a newer, riskier technique called 'whole genome shotgun sequencing', which had previously been used in the sequencing of bacterial genomes.

- Although the working draft was announced in June 2000, it was not until February 2001 that Celera and the HGP scientists published actual details of their drafts.

7

- – Special issues of *Nature* (which published the publicly funded project's scientific paper) and *Science* (which published Celera's paper) contained descriptions of the methods used to produce the draft sequence, as well as an analysis of the sequence.

- The information provided by the HGP (which is available to the public) is expected to have a great impact in the diagnostics and treatment of cancer.
  - – The great advances made in basic science in the last 20 years are already having an impact on speeding the rate of drug discovery in the field of cancer, giving many reasons for hope and optimism to those who choose to fight this relentless disease.

2

Epidemiology of prostate cancer

Worldwide

[Parkin DM, CA Cancer J Clin **55**: 74–108, 2005]
[Ferlay J, Globocan 2002: Cancer Incidence, Mortality and Prevalence Worldwide. IARC CancerBase No. 5, version 2.0. International Agency for Research on Cancer, Lyon, 2004]
[Parkin DM, Cancer in Five Continents. IARC Scientific Publications No. 155. International Agency for Research on Cancer, Lyon, 2003]

- Globally, prostate cancer is the fifth most common cancer, with 679,023 new prostate cancer cases diagnosed yearly and 221,002 deaths/year.

- Prostate cancer is a disease with strong geographic variation, both internationally and also within individual countries and regions.

- Prostate cancer is the second most common cancer in ♂, accounting for 11.7% of new cancer cases overall.
  - 19% in developed countries.
  - 5.3% in developing countries.

- The worldwide 5-year prevalence of prostate cancer has been estimated at 2,368,659.
  - 83% of these cases are in the developed countries.

- The incidence of prostate cancer varies from country to country.
  - The highest rates occur in North America, Europe, and Australia/ New Zealand.

- The lowest rates reported are in Asia, most of Africa, and the Middle East.
- The age-adjusted incidence rate in the USA is 124.8/100,000 vs 1.7/100,000 and 12.6/100,000 in China and Japan, respectively.

- \> 70% of all prostate cancer cases are diagnosed in ♂ aged > 65 years.

- The number of new cases ↑ rapidly in the 1990s.
  - This was largely because of the greater use of the prostate-specific antigen (PSA) test, which led to more cases of prostate cancer being detected.

- Survival is significantly better in high-risk countries: ratio of age-standardized rates (incidence and death) is 87% in the USA vs 45% in developing countries.

- Mortality rates are high in the Caribbean, southern and central Africa, north and west Europe, Australia/New Zealand, and the USA, and low in Asia populations and north Africa.

North America

[American Cancer Society, *Cancer Facts and Figures – 2005*. American Cancer Society, Atlanta, GA, 2005]
[Ries LAG, *SEER Cancer Statistics Review, 1975–2002*. National Cancer Institute, Bethesda, MD, 2005]
[Haas GP, *CA Cancer J Clin* **47**: 272–287, 1997]

New cases

- The American Cancer Society predicted that, in 2005, ~ 232,090 new cases of prostate cancer would be diagnosed in the USA.

- 1/6 American ♂ will be diagnosed with prostate cancer in his lifetime.
  - The lifetime probability of being diagnosed with prostate cancer is 8%.

- The incidence of prostate cancer varies by US state.
  - States estimated to have the largest numbers of new cases in 2005 were California, Florida, New York, Texas, and Pennsylvania.
  - Migrants from low-risk countries to areas of ↑ risk show a quite marked ↑ in incidence.

- African American and Jamaican ♂ of African descent have the highest prostate cancer incidence rates in the world,

- – Rates are ∼ 70% higher in blacks than whites.
- Asian origin, like Chinese, Japanese, and Korean, has ↓ rates than whites.
  - – Japanese living in the USA have ↑ rates than Japanese living in Japan.
- These results strongly suggest that environmental factors contribute to the large differences in risk found between countries.
- Between 1975 and 1992 prostate cancer rates ↑ dramatically.
  - – Partly due to a genuine ↑ in risk.
  - – ↑ life expectancy.
  - – Partly due to ↑ diagnosis of latent, asymptomatic cancers in prostatectomy specimens resulting from the ↑ use of transurethral resection of the prostate.
  - – To earlier diagnosis because of PSA blood tests.
- Prostate cancer rates subsequently ↓ and have ↑ at less rapid rates since 1995 due to the ↑ rate in ♂ aged < 65 years, probably due to widespread screening with the PSA test.
- In those aged ≥ 65 years, however, rates have leveled off.
  - – Rates peaked in 1992 among white ♂ (237.5/100,000) and in 1993 among African American ♂ (341.4/100,000).

Deaths

- With an estimated 30,350 deaths in 2005, prostate cancer is the second leading cause of cancer death in ♂.
- Since the early 1990s, death rates have been ↓ among white and African American ♂.
  - – Patients are more frequently diagnosed with localized disease (53% in 1986 compared with 74% in 1996) and ↓ grade tumors.
  - – Rates in African American ♂ remain > 2× the rates in white ♂.

Survival

- 5-year survival rates.
  - – Early-stage prostate cancer: ∼ 100%.
  - – Late stage prostate cancer: 33.5%.
- 10-year survival rate for all prostate cancer patients: 92%.
- 15-year survival rate for all prostate cancer patients: 61%.

- 5-year survival rate ↑ for all prostate cancer patients over the past 20 years: from 67% to 99%.
  - The dramatic improvements in survival, particularly at 5 years, are partly attributable to earlier diagnosis and to some improvements in treatment.

Age distribution

- The incidence of prostate cancer ↑ with age.
  - There are virtually no cases in ♂ aged < 40 years, and rates are highest among ♂ aged 70–74 years.
- In 1998–2002 the age-specific rate among ♂ aged 40–44 years was 8.5/100,000, whereas that in ♂ aged 70–74 years was 1,096/100,000.

Africa

[Parkin DM, *Cancer in Africa: Epidemiology and Prevention*. International Agency for Research on Cancer, Lyon, 2003, pp. 362–366]

- Comparability of statistics on the incidence of prostate cancer is hampered by different practices concerning:
  - Biopsy of lesions.
  - The extent of histological examination of biopsy material.
  - The use of the PSA test for diagnosis.

- Unlike in North America and Europe, a diagnosed case in Africa almost always implies a clinically evident, frankly invasive, relatively advanced tumor.

- The incidence of prostate cancer varies greatly between the different regions of Africa.
  - It is difficult to be sure whether the regional variations seen are real or simply reflect awareness of the disease and diagnostic capabilities.
  - Incidence rates appear to be low in all the countries of North Africa.
  - Rates appear to be ↑ in urban populations than in rural settings.
    - Incidence rates are ↑ in cities such as Abidjan (Cote d'Ivoire) and Harare (Zimbabwe).
  - Rates are ↑ in white populations than in black ones.
    - This probably represents the more ready access of whites to modern diagnostic and treatment methods, as well as to PSA testing.

- Incidence rates in the more recent series are ↑ than those reported in the past.

The UK and Europe

[Cancer Research UK, Cancer Stats UK, 2004. http://info.cancer researchuk.org]
[Cancer Research UK, Statistics: Mortality, 2004. http://info.cancer researchuk.org]
[Cancer Research UK, Men's Cancers Factsheet, 2005. http://info. cancer researchuk.org]
[Boyle P, Ann Oncol 16: 481–488, 2005]
[Grulich AE, Br J Cancer 66: 905–911, 1992]
[Bouchardy C, Int J Epidemiol 6: 539–534, 1990]
[Shimizu H, Br J Cancer 63(6): 963–966, 1991]
[Tsugane S, Int J Cancer 45(3): 436–439, 1990]

- Prostate cancer is the most common cancer in ♂ in the UK, being responsible for a fifth of all new cancer cases.
  - Over 30,000 new cases a year.
  - > 80% of cases are diagnosed in ♂ > 65 years old.
  - Lifetime risk for being diagnosed with prostate cancer is 1 in 14.

- The overall incidence of prostate cancer is 98/100,000.
  - Ranging from 5.8/100,000 in ♂ aged 45–49 years.
  - To 945.8/100,000 in ♂ aged > 85 years.

- Prostate cancer is the second largest cause of death.
  - > 10,000 deaths reported in 2003.
  - Accounting for ~ 13% of cancer deaths in ♂.
  - ~ 85% of deaths are in ♂ > 70 years old.

- The overall mortality rate is 35/100,000.
  - Ranging from 2/100,000 in ♂ aged 45–54 years.
  - To 846/100,000 in ♂ aged > 85 years.

- Between 1975 and 2001 the age-adjusted incidence rate doubled, while the age-adjusted mortality did not change significantly.

- The 1-and 5-year survival rates have improved significantly since the 1970s.
  - 1-year survival: 65% in 1971–1975; 87% in 1996–1999.
  - 5-year survival: 31% in 1971–1975; 65% in 1996–1999.

- In 2004 in Europe, prostate cancer was the second most frequent form of cancer in ♂.
  - 237,800 new cases and 85,200 deaths.
  - 15.5% of new cancer cases; 8.9% of all cancer-related deaths
  - The age-standardized incidence was 65/100,000, and mortality was 26/100,000 in 2003.

- Migrants from West Africa and the Caribbean to England and Wales have significantly ↑ mortality rates than those of the local-born population; in contrast, the mortality among migrants from East Africa, of predominantly Asian (Indian) ethnicity, is not high.

- In keeping with the low rates of prostate cancer in their countries of origin, migrants to France from North Africa (Morocco, Algeria, and Tunisia) had significantly ↓ mortality rates than local-born ♂.
  - These results contradict other data showing that when individuals from a low incidence/mortality region move to a high incidence/mortality region the disease becomes more common.
  - The incidence among Japanese ♂ living in Los Angeles County was ↑ than among those living in Japan.
  - A significantly ↑ standardized mortality ratio was reported among Japan-born residents of Sao Paulo, Brazil, compared with residents of Japan.
  - It is clear that the effect of relocation depends on the age at the time of relocation and the length of time living in the new environment.

Asia

[Sim HG, *Eur J Cancer* **41**(6): 834–845, 2005]
[Sasagawa I, *Arch Androl* **47**(3): 195–201, 2001]

- There has been a recent trend in Asia towards ↑ incidence of prostate cancer, with some low-risk regions, such as Japan and Singapore, reporting a more rapid ↑ than high-risk countries.
  - Incidence in some parts of Japan rose from 6.3/100,000 to 12.7/100,000.
  - The incidence in Singaporean Chinese ↑ from 6.6/100,000 to 14.4/100,000 person-years.
  - These incidences are still much ↓ than those in the USA and many European countries.

- The mortality data for prostate cancer showed a similar trend.
  - In Japan, between 1980 and 1998, the age-adjusted death rates due to prostate cancer ↑ from 4.4/100,000 to 8.6/100,000.

3

Risk factors

[Bostwick DG, *Cancer* **101**: 2371–2400, 2004]
[Gronberg H, *Lancet* **361**: 859–864, 2003]

Factors that increase risk

Age

- The prostate may be the most disease-prone organ of the human body with aging.

- Frequencies of benign prostatic hyperplasia and prostate cancer ↑ dramatically with age, beginning with low frequencies in middle-aged ♂ and progressing to > 90% by age 90 years.

- 1 in 48 ♂ aged 40–59 years will be diagnosed with prostate cancer.

- 1 in 8 ♂ aged 60–79 years are at risk.
  [*DevCan: Probability of Developing or Dying of Cancer*. National Cancer Institute, Bethesda, MD. Available at: http://srab.cancer.gov/devcan (accessed 9 August 2007)]
  [Coffey DS, *Urol Clin North Am* **17**: 461–475, 1990]

- With aging there is a progressive accumulation of DNA damage, likely caused by oxidative stress, due to an imbalance in cellular pro-oxidant–antioxidant status.
  [He P, *Mech Aging Dev* **76**: 43–48, 1994]

Race

- Race-related differences in prostate-cancer risk may reflect multiple factors, including exposure differences, particularly dietary differences, differences in detection, and genetic differences.

- The estimated lifetime risk of disease is 16.6% for caucasians and 18.1% for African Americans. The lifetime risk of death is 3.5% and 4.3%, respectively.

- African American ♂ have a 65% greater risk of developing prostate cancer than Caucasian ♂.

- ↓ risk for Asian/Pacific Islander and Hispanic American ♂ compared with caucasian American ♂.
  [*DevCan: Probability of Developing or Dying of Cancer.* National Cancer Institute, Bethesda, MD. Available at: http://srab.cancer.gov/devcan (accessed 9 August 2007)]

- African American ♂ in the USA are more likely to present with advanced stage cancers than white ♂, and their stage-specific mortality is worse, especially among younger ♂.
  [Hoffman RM, *J Natl Cancer Inst* **93**: 388–395, 2001]

- African American and Hispanic ♂ are commonly diagnosed at a significantly younger average age (mean 63.7 and 65.2 years, respectively) compared with white ♂ (mean 68.1 years).
  [Cotter MP, *Prostate* **50**: 216–221, 2002]

- African American ♂ have a higher intake of dietary fat, and this may contribute to their higher risk.
  [Whittemore AS, *J Natl Cancer Inst* **87**: 652–661, 1995]

- Some of the differences in risk between black and white Americans may reflect their access to healthcare.
  [Haas GP, *CA Cancer J Clin* **47**: 273–287, 1997]

- There are racial differences in allelic frequencies of the androgen receptor (AR) locus and other genes, which may promote prostate cell growth, resulting in ↑ prostate cancer risk for African American ♂.
  [Platz EA, *J Natl Cancer Inst* **92**: 2009–2017, 2000]

- Sex-hormone-binding globulin levels are ↑ in young, adult African Americans, and this may contribute to a subsequent ↑ risk of prostate cancer.

- The activity of 5-α-reductase is lower among Japanese ♂ than among African American and white ♂.
  [Ross RK, *Lancet* **339**: 887–889, 1992]

Family history

- Prostate cancer appears to have a stronger familial aggregation than colon or breast cancer.
  [Carter BS, *J Urol* **50**: 797–802, 1993]

- A patient with a first-degree relative with prostate cancer is 2.4 times as likely to be diagnosed with prostate cancer as a ♂ with no affected relatives.
  [Neal DE, *Eur J Cancer* **36**: 1316–1321, 2000]

- ♂ with 3 first-degree or second-degree affected relatives have a ×11 greater risk of developing prostate cancer.
  [Steinberg GD, *Prostate* **17**: 337–347, 1990]

- Twin studies showed that this risk is based, in part, on a shared genetic predisposition.
  [Gronberg H, *J Urol* **152**: 1484–1487, 1994]

- The rate of prostate cancer is greater among monozygotic (27.1%) than dizygotic twin pairs (7.1%).
  [Page WF, *Prostate* **33**: 240–245, 1997]

- Risk is ↑ with greater genetic linkage of a ♂ to an affected relative, and with the greater number of relatives he has with prostate cancer.
  [Eeles RA, *Prostate Cancer Prostatic Dis* **2**: 9–15, 1999]

- Family history predicts an ↑ risk for aggressive prostate cancer.
  [Klein EA, *Prostate Cancer Prostatic Dis* **1**: 297–300, 1998]

- Several studies have reported an ↑ prostate cancer risk among ♂ with first-degree ♀ relatives who had breast cancer, but others failed to find this association.
  [Cerhan JR, *Cancer Epidemiol Biomarker Prev* **8**: 53–60, 1999]

Hormones

- ↑ levels of testosterone and its metabolite dihydrotestosterone, over many decades, may ↑ prostate cancer risk.

- Paradoxically, serum testosterone levels are declining in ♂ at the age of peak cancer incidence.
  [Henderson BE, *Cancer Res* **42**: 3232–3239, 1982]

- The absence of an association between plasma levels of androgens and prostate cancer risk may be a result of the complex and inverse associations of androgenicity to insulin-like growth factor I (IGF-I), insulin, and leptin.

- IGF regulates proliferation, differentiation, and apoptosis of cancer cells; ↑ concentrations of IGF are associated with ↑ risk of prostate cancer. [Kaaks R, *Eur J Cancer Prev* **12**: 309–315, 2003]

- Leptin influences cellular differentiation and the progression of prostate cancer through testosterone and through factors related to obesity.

- ♂ with high-volume cancer had higher leptin concentrations at the time of prostate cancer diagnosis. [Saglam K, *J Urol* **169**: 1308–1311, 2003] [Chang S, *Prostate* **46**: 62–67, 2001]

Hereditary prostate cancer

- Both familial and hereditary prostate cancers are diagnosed approximately 6–7 years earlier than the sporadic form of the disease.

- Studies suggest that the disease in these patients does not, for the most part, differ in clinical presentation, response to treatment, or survival. [Valeri A, *Prostate* **5**: 66–71, 2000] [Bratt O, *J Urol* **167**: 2423–2426, 2000]

Androgen receptor

[Brinkmann AO, *J Steroid Biochem Mol Biol* **40**: 349–352, 1991] [Tilley WD, *Cancer Res* **50**: 5382–5386, 1990]

- The AR plays a crucial role in prostate cancer.

- AR blockade can delay the progression of prostate cancer, and is used to treat patients unsuitable for radical surgery or with cancer that has spread beyond the prostate.

- Androgens are required for the development of both the normal prostate and prostate cancer.

- Initially, most prostate cancers are sensitive to androgen deprivation.

- In patients with advanced disease, most tumors progress to an androgen-independent state.

- The mechanism of acquired androgen insensitivity is unknown.

- Mutations, amplifications, and deletions of the AR gene and structural changes in the AR protein have been postulated to cause androgen insensitivity.

- Structural change of the AR has been identified in only a minority of androgen-insensitive prostate cancers

CYP17

[Chang B, *Int J Cancer* **95**: 354–359, 2001]
[Standord JL, *Cancer Epidemiol Biomarkers Prev* **11**: 243–247, 2002]

- Encodes cytochrome P450c17α, an enzyme responsible for the biosynthesis of testosterone.
- A variant CYP17 allele is associated with both hereditary and sporadic prostate cancer.
- Hypothesized to ↑ the rate of gene transcription, ↑ androgen production, and thereby ↑ the risk of prostate cancer.

SRD5A2

[Makridakis NM, *Lancet* **354**: 975–978, 1999]

- Encodes the predominant isozyme of 5-α-reductase in the prostate, an enzyme that converts testosterone to the more potent dihydrotestosterone.
- Alleles that encode enzymes with ↑ activity have been associated with an ↑ risk of prostate cancer, and with a poor prognosis for ♂ with prostate cancer.

HPC1/RNASEL

[Wang L, *Am J Hum Genet* **71**: 116–123, 2002]
[Nakazato H, *Br J Cancer* **89**: 691–696, 2003]

- Ribonuclease that degrades viral and cellular RNA and can produce apoptosis on viral infection.
- Mutations have been identified in familial and sporadic prostate cancer in many studies, although other studies have not supported these findings.
- There is strong support that *RNASEL* is the most important hereditary prostate cancer gene identified to date.

HPC2/ELAC2

[Rebbeck TR, *Am J Hum Genet* **61**: 1014–1019, 2000]
[Suarez BK, *Cancer Res* **61**: 4982–4984, 2001]

- The first possible hereditary prostate cancer gene to be identified.

- Its function is not known; proposed as a metal-dependent hydrolase.
- Association with familial prostate cancer has been reported.
- Has a minor role in prostate cancer.

Retinoblastoma

[Brooks JD, *Prostate* **26**: 35–39, 1995]

- Disruption of the normal retinoblastoma (Rb) regulatory pathway is associated with the pathogenesis of many human cancers.
- The *Rb* gene plays an important role in the G1 phase of the cell cycle.
- Rb protein binds tightly to the E2F family of transcription factors.
  - When phosphorylated, the Rb protein releases the E2F proteins, causing transcriptional activation of a variety of genes involved in cell growth.

p53

[Gao X, *Prostate* **31**: 264–281, 1997]

- Low frequency of mutation of this gene in prostate cancer.
- Abnormal *p53* expression is associated with bone metastases and the development of androgen-independent disease.
- Correlates with high histologic grade, high stage, clinical disease progression, and ↓ survival.
- *p53* tumor suppressor gene product restricts entry into the synthetic phase of the cell cycle and promotes apoptosis in cells that have damaged DNA.
- Loss of normal *p53* function results in uncontrolled cell growth.

c-myc

[Jenkin RB, *Cancer Res* **57**: 524–531, 1997]

- Increased expression in prostate cancer.
- Significant correlation between *myc* overexpression and Gleason grade.
- Myc proteins act as transcriptional factors.

bcl-2

[Catz SD, *Apoptosis* **8**: 29–37, 2003]

- Commonly expressed in primary and metastatic prostate cancers.
- Plays a crucial role in the regulation of apotosis.
- Implicated in the development of androgen-independent prostate cancer.

c-Kit/tyrosine kinase receptor

[Paronetto MP, *Am J Pathol* **164**: 1243–1251, 2004]

- Strong activator of the Src family of tyrosine kinases.
- tr-Kit mRNA and protein are expressed in prostatic cancer cells.

MSR1

[Dejager S, *J Clin Invest* **92**: 894 902, 1993]
[Wang L, *Nat Genet* **35**: 128–129, 2003]

- Encodes a macrophage scavenger receptor responsible for cellular uptake of molecules, including bacterial cell-wall products.
- Germline *MSR1* mutations have been linked to prostate cancer in some families with prostate cancer and in sporadic prostate cancer.
  - However, other studies did not provide confirmatory evidence of the role of *MSR1* in familial prostate cancer.
- Mutations of these host responses to infection genes may ↑ the risk of prostate cancer by predisposing to chronic inflammation as a result of failure of viral RNA and bacterial degradation.

Nijmegen breakage syndrome (NBS1 gene)

[Demuth I, *Hum Mol Genet* **13**: 2385–2397, 2004]
[Cybulski C, *Cancer Res* **64**: 1215–1219, 2004]

- Rare genetic disorder.
- Characterized by radiosensitivity, immunodeficiency, chromosomal instability, and an ↑ risk of cancer of the lymphatic system.
- *NBS1* encodes a protein, nibrin, involved in the processing/repair of DNA double-strand breaks and in cell-cycle checkpoints.

- Mutations have been identified in both sporadic and familial cases of prostate cancer.

- Associated with a small ↑ risk of prostate cancer.

CHEK2

[Dong XA, *J Hum Genet* **72**: 270–280, 2003]

- Upstream regulator of *p53* in the DNA damage signaling pathway.

- Mutations identified in both sporadic and familial cases of prostate cancer.

- Small ↑ risk of prostate cancer.

TLR4

[Zheng SL, *Cancer Res* **64**: 2918–2922, 2004]

- Encodes a receptor that is a central player in the signaling pathways of the innate immune response to infection by Gram-negative bacteria.

- A sequence polymorphism is associated with a small ↑ risk of prostate cancer.

Vitamin D receptor

[Skowronski RJ, *Endocrinology* **132**: 1952–1960, 1993]

- Physiological concentrations of vitamin D promote the differentiation and growth arrest of prostate cancer cells in vitro.

- Precise mechanism unknown, but probably acts through its effect on cell-growth proteins.

- Vitamin D receptor alleles have been associated with prostate cancer.

Glutathione S-transferase gene (GSTP1)

[Millar DS, *Oncogene* **18**: 1313–1324, 1999]
[Harden SV, *J Urol* **169**: 1138–1142, 2003]

- One of the most important tumor suppressor genes in prostate cancer.

- GSTP1 can detoxify environmental carcinogens and oxidants and may play a genome caretaker role by preventing DNA damage.

- GSTP1 has been shown to be inactivated by hypermethylation in prostate tumors.

- This is the most common (> 90%) reported epigenetic alteration in prostate cancer.

- Occurs early in cancer progression, and is a promising marker for detecting organ-confined disease.

- Quantitation of GSTP1 hypermethylation can accurately detect the presence of cancer, even in small, limited tissue samples.
    - Could possibly be used as an adjunct to tissue biopsy as part of screening for prostate cancer.

PTEN (phosphatase and tensin homolog)

[Suzuki H, Cancer Res 58: 204–209, 1998]

- An important tumor-suppressor gene in prostate cancer.

- Influences the concentrations of CDKN1B, another important tumor-suppressor gene.

- Common target for somatic changes during the progression of prostate cancer.

- In prostate cancers, concentrations of PTEN are often reduced, particularly in cancers of high grade or stage.

CDKN1B (p27)

[Chang BL, Cancer Res 64: 1997–1999, 2004]
[Cote RJ, J Natl Cancer Inst 90: 916–920, 1998]
[Kibel AS, J Urol 164: 192–196, 2000]

- Functions as an important cell-cycle gatekeeper.

- Association between a single nucleotide polymorphism of CDKN1B (p27) and prostate cancer.

- An important tumor-suppressor gene in prostate cancer.

- Reduced concentrations of p27, a cyclin-dependent kinase inhibitor encoded by the CDKN1B gene, are common in prostate cancers, particularly in those with a poor prognosis.

- Somatic loss of DNA sequences encompassing CDKN1B.
    - Has been described in 23% of localized prostate cancers, 30% of

prostate cancer metastases in regional lymph nodes, and 47% of distant prostate cancer metastases.

Other genes and signaling pathways alterations

[Hughes C, *J Clin Pathol* **58**: 673–684, 2005]

- Ongoing research regarding new genes and signaling pathway alterations, including, but not limited to, *NKX3.1*, *KLF6*, *STAT5*, hepsin, α-methylacyl coenzyme A racemase (AMACR) gene, *PIM1*, *MTA1*, *EZH2*, *C-erb 2* (*Her-2 neu*), *c-met*, and *Fas/Fas* ligand.

- Prostate cancer is probably caused by multiple genes with complex interactions.

- Many studies have concentrated on one gene at a time.

- Future studies may need to consider the simultaneous effects of multiple genes.

Estimating risk factors

[Zeegers MP, *Cancer* **97**: 1894–1903, 2003]
[Glover FE, *Urology* **52**: 441–443, 1998]
[Gronberg H, *Cancer* **86**: 477–483, 1999]
[Aprikian AG, *J Urol* **54**: 404–406, 1995]
[Lesko SM, *Am J Epidemiol* **144**: 1041–1047, 1996]

- The risk of developing prostate cancer ↑ with the number of affected ♂ relatives.

- A ♂ with one first-degree relative affected by prostate cancer is twice as likely as ♂ in the general population to develop prostate cancer.

- If his relatives develop prostate cancer at an earlier age, the risk ↑ further.

- If two or more first-degree relatives are affected at an early age (< 65 years), the risk is ↑ ×4 (Table 3.1).

- The cumulative risks for ♂ with two affected first-degree relatives simulates an autosomal-dominant trait.

- For African American ♂ the risks of developing prostate cancer based on ethnicity alone are 40–80% greater than for caucasian ♂.

- Although the baseline risks for developing prostate cancer are different, the familial risks do not vary with ethnicity.

- The net effect of a family history of prostate cancer is to make the risk for younger ♂ with a positive family history comparable to that for older ♂ without a family history.

- The net effect of ethnicity is to make the risks for younger African American ♂ comparable to that for older caucasian ♂.
  [Zeegers MP, *Cancer* **97**: 1894–1903, 2003]
  [Carter BS, *Proc Natl Acad Sci USA* **89**: 3367–3371, 1992]
  [Gronberg H, *Am J Epidemiol* **146**: 552–557, 1997]

Genetic testing

[Ostrander EA, *Am J Hum Genet* **67**: 1367–1375, 2000].
[Nieder AM, *Clin Genet* **63**: 169–176, 2003]

- Linkage analysis of ♂ from high-risk families has led to the identification of multiple susceptibility loci.

- Within some populations, the high-risk loci might account for a significant proportion of cases of prostate cancer.
  - However, this appears to be the exception rather than the rule, because a major problem with linkage studies has been the difficulty of replicating findings across populations with hereditary prostate cancer.

- It is not clear which genetic tests, if any, should be offered to a ♂ with a single first-degree relative affected by prostate cancer by age 55 years.

- Genetic counseling of ♂ at ↑ risk of prostate cancer should include a detailed family history of the diagnosis and age of onset of prostate and other cancers in family members.

- From the pedigree analysis, an age-related risk estimate can be provided to gauge when screening for prostate cancer should be offered.

- ♂ with multiple affected relatives should be offered participation in a research study.

Current recommendations for high-risk patients

- The American Urological Association recommends that in ♂ at higher risk of prostate cancer, based on family history or ethnicity, screening should start at age 40 years.
  [Carroll P, *Urology* **57**: 217–224, 2001]

Table 3.1 Cumulative risk of developing prostate cancer, by age, family history, and ethnicity

	Relative risk	Cumulative risk (%) by age (95% CI)			
		40 years	50 years	60 years	70 years
White men					
No family history	1	0.005	0.162	2.04	7.5
One first-degree relative	2.57 (2.32–2.84)	0.013 (0.012–0.014)	0.416 (0.376–0.460)	5.24 (4.73–5.79)	19.28 (17.40–21.30)
Family member diagnosed < 65 years old	3.34 (2.64–4.23)	0.017 (0.013–0.021)	0.541 (0.428–0.685)	6.81 (5.39–8.63)	25.05 (19.80–31.73)
Family member diagnosed ≥ 65 years old	2.35 (2.05–2.70)	0.012 (0.010–0.014)	0.381 (0.332–0.437)	4.79 (4.18–5.51)	17.63 (15.38–20.25)
Two or more first-degree relatives	5.08 (3.31–7.79)	0.025 (0.017–0.039)	0.832 (0.536–1.26)	10.36 (6.75–15.89)	38.10 (24.83–58.43)
Second-degree relative	1.68 (1.07–2.64)	0.008 (0.005–0.013)	0.272 (0.173–0.428)	3.43 (2.18–5.39)	12.60 (8.03–19.80)

Black men

No family history	1	0.009	0.417	3.589	10.549
One first-degree relative	2.57 (2.52–2.84)	0.023 (0 021–0.026)	1.07 (0.97–1.18)	9.22 (8.33–10.19)	27.11 (24.47–29.96)
Family member < 65 years old diagnosed	3.34 (2.63–4.23)	0.030 (0 024–0.038)	1.39 (1.10–1.76)	11.99 (9.44–15.18)	35.23 (27.74–44.62)
Family member diagnosed ≥ 65 years old	2.35 (2.05–2.70)	0.021 (0.019–0.024)	0.98 (0.86–1.13)	8.43 (7.36–9.69)	24.79 (21.63–28.48)
Two or more first-degree relatives	5.08 (3.31–7.79)	0.046 (0.030–0.071)	2.12 (1.38–3.25)	18.23 (11.88–27.96)	33.59 (34.52–82.018)
Second-degree relative	1.68 (1.07–2.64)	0.015 (0.010–0.024)	0.70 (0.45–1.10)	6.03 (3.84–9.47)	17.72 (11.29–27.85)

[Nieder AM, *Clin Genet* 63: 169–176, 2003]

- The American Cancer Society recommends that screening starts at age 45 years for African American ♂ and for ♂ with one affected first-degree relative, and at age 40 years for ♂ at higher risk.
  [Smith RA, CA Cancer J Clin **52**: 8–22, 2002]

- However, the American College of Physicians and the American College of Preventative Medicine do not recommend the use of routine screening.
  [American College of Physicians, Ann Intern Med **126**: 480–484, 1997]

- Even in the absence of genetic testing, African American ♂ and ♂ with a strong family history of prostate cancer may opt to initiate screening by prostate specific antigen (PSA) and digital rectal examination at age 40 years.

- African American ♂ with prostate cancer tend to have a more aggressive form of the disease compared with other ethnic groups.
  - Younger age.
  - Higher stage of disease.
  - Higher Gleason scores.
  - Higher mean PSAs.
  - ↓ response to therapy.

- African American ♂ had a significantly ↑ percentage of positive biopsies when matched with their white counterparts for PSA level.

- No difference in treatment is justified exclusively on the basis of family history.
  [Hanus MC, Int J Radiat Oncol Biol Phys **43**: 379–383, 1999]
  [Gronberg H, JAMA **278**: 1251–1255, 1997]
  [Lubeck DP, J Urol **166**: 2281–2285, 2001]
  [Carvalhal GF, J Urol **162**: 113–118, 1999]

Potential risk factors

Vasectomy

- Moderately ↑ risk of prostate cancer.
  [Lightfoot N, Ann Epidemiol **10**: 470, 2000]

- ↑ in risk has been reported to be in the range 1.5–2.0.
  [Mettlin C, Am J Epidemiol **132**: 1056–1061, 1990]

- Relationship remains controversial because other studies have found no association.
  [Nienhuis H, BMJ **304**: 743–746, 1992]

Chronic prostatitis

[De Marzo AM, *Am J Pathol* **92**: 1985–1992, 1999]

- Chronic inflammation may contribute to prostate carcinogenesis.

- Focal prostatic glandular atrophy, suggested as a potential precursor to prostatic adenocarcinoma, is closely associated with chronic inflammation.

Obesity

[Amling CL, *Curr Opinion Urol* **15**: 167–171, 2005]
[Bergstrom A, *Int J Cancer* **91**: 421–430, 2001]

- ↓ Leptin = ↑ obesity = ↑ prostate cancer.

- Obesity linked to aggressiveness and recurrence of prostate cancer.

- Obesity and being overweight ↑ the risk of prostate cancer by 12% and 6%, respectively.

Diet

- Strong, positive correlation (0.74) between prostate cancer incidence or mortality and fat consumption, in multiple countries.
  [Howell MA, *Br J Cancer* **29**: 328–336, 1979]

- ↑ risk attributable to high levels of saturated fat intake.
  [Kolonel LN, *Epidemiol Rev* **23**: 72–81, 2001]

Smoking

[Hickey K, *Epidemiol Rev* **23**: 115–125, 2001]

- The association between current smoking and prostate cancer is controversial.

- Cadmium is thought to be present in tobacco smoke, and laboratory studies found some evidence to support a role of cadmium in prostate cancer.

- Mutation in the tumor suppressor gene *p53* may be a mechanism that explains the association between smoking and fatal prostate cancer.

Alcohol

- No ↑ or ↓ risk associated with alcohol intake.
  [Andersson SO, *Int J Cancer* **68**: 716–722, 1996]

Factors that decrease risk

Cirrhosis

- ↑ estrogen levels, severe enough to lead to testicular atrophy and ↓ risk of prostate cancer.
  [Glantz GM, *J Urol* **91**: 291–293, 1964]

Diabetes mellitus

[Adami HO, *Cancer Causes Control* **2**: 307–314, 1991]
[Ando S, *J Endocrinol* **7**: 21–24, 1984]
[Giovannucci E, *Cancer Causes Control* **9**: 3–9, 1998]

- ↓ prostate cancer risk by 30–70% among ♂ with type II diabetes mellitus.

- Risk appears to ↓ over time since diagnosis of diabetes.

- ↓ androgen levels, probably resulting from the toxic effects of hyperglycemia on the testosterone-producing Leydig cells.
    - ↓ total and free testosterone levels are among the numerous metabolic and hormonal aberrations associated with diabetes.

Finasteride

[Thompson PJ, *N Engl J Med* **349**: 215–224, 2003]

- Associated with a 25% overall ↓ in prostate cancer prevalence.

- ↑ incidence of high-grade cancers were more common with finasteride compared to placebo.

Selenium

[Klein EA, *J Urol* **171**: S50–S53, 2004]
[Duffield-Lillico AJ, *Br J Urol* **91**: 608–612, 2003]

- Case–control and randomized placebo-controlled trials in humans suggest that selenium can ↓ risk of getting prostate cancer.

- Selenium inhibits tumorigenesis in a variety of experimental models.

- ↓ incidence of prostate cancer in those receiving selenium by two-thirds compared with placebo.

Zinc

[Haas GP, *CA Cancer J Clin* **47**: 273–287, 1997]
[Feustel A, *Prostate* **8**: 75–79, 1986]

- The prostate has a higher concentration of zinc than any other organ in the human body.

- The physiologic role of zinc in the prostate is unknown.

- Cancer-bearing prostates have lower levels of zinc compared with non-cancer-bearing prostates.

Alpha-Tocopherol, Beta-Carotene Cancer Prevention Trial (ATBC Trial)

[Ni J, *Biochem Biophys Res Commun* **300**: 357–363, 2003]
[Virtamo J, *JAMA* **290**: 476–485, 2003]

- Vitamin E modulates prostate cancer cell growth by causing G1 cell-cycle arrest.
  - It ↓ expression of the cell-cycle regulatory proteins cyclin D1, D3, and E, and cdk2 and cdk4.

- This supports the role of vitamin E in the prevention of prostate cancer.

- There is a statistically significant 32% ↓ in prostate cancer incidence and a 41% ↓ in mortality in those receiving α-tocopherol.

- Effects washout after discontinuation of treatment, which has an important implication on the need for long-term use of dietary supplements to prevent cancer.

Vitamin D

[Krishnan AV, *J Cell Biochem* **88**: 363–371, 2003]

- Microarray gene expression studies demonstrate that active vitamin D exerts its antiproliferative activity by inducing cell-cycle arrest.
  - This is mediated by induction of IGF binding protein-3 expression, which ↑ levels of the cell-cycle inhibitor p21.

- Use of vitamin D is limited by its hypercalcemic effects.

Non-steroidal anti-inflammatory drugs

[Pruthi RS, *J Urol* **169**: 2352–2359, 2003]
[Hussain T, *Cancer Lett* **191**: 125–135, 2003]

- Non-steroidal anti-inflammatory drugs (NSAIDs) block proinflammatory effects and may underlie an important anticancer mechanism.

- ↑ expression of COX-2 is known to correlate with ↑ angiogenesis, ↓ apoptosis, and ↑ tumor invasiveness and immunosuppression.

- Prostate cancer expresses more COX-2, and several epidemiologic studies have noted an inverse association between prostate cancer and the use of NSAIDs.

Soy

[Lee MM, *Cancer Epidemiol Biomarkers Prev* **12**: 665–668, 2003]
[Hedlund TE, *Prostate* **54**: 68–78, 2003]
[Wang S, *J Nutr* **133**: 2367–2376, 2003]

- A case–control study in China demonstrated a marked protective effect against prostate cancer of both tofu and soy consumption.

- The major isoflavone components of soy inhibit benign and malignant prostatic epithelial cell growth, down-regulate androgen-regulated genes, and reduce tumor growth in animal models.

- Recent studies suggest these effects are mediated in part by inhibition of IGF-I, resulting in cell-cycle arrest and induction of apoptosis, and by proteasome inhibition.

Lycopene

[Obermuller-Jevic UC, *J Nutr* **133**: 3356–3360, 2003]

- A carotenoid found primarily in tomatoes, lycopene is a highly unsaturated acyclic isomer of β-carotene, and possesses potent antioxidant activity.

- It inhibits the growth of benign and malignant prostatic epithelial cells.

- There is mixed epidemiologic evidence that lycopene is associated with a ↓ risk of prostate cancer.

Green tea

[Adhami VM, *J Nutr* **133**: 2417S–2424S, 2003]

- There is a low incidence of prostate cancer among native Asians with a high dietary intake of green tea.

- The major polyphenolic constituent of green tea induces apoptosis, cell-growth inhibition, and cycline kinase inhibitor WAF-1/p21-mediated cell-cycle dysregulation in prostate cancer cell culture experiments.

Chemoprevention

[Klein EA, *Crit Rev Oncol Hematol* **54**: 1–10, 2005]
[Gupta S, *Int J Oncol* **25**: 1133–1148, 2004]
[Fujimoto N, *Urol Int* **74**: 289–297, 2005]
[Mahal K, *Curr Urol Rep* **6**: 177–182, 2005]

- There is no recommended agent, vitamin, or nutritional supplement that has been shown to prevent prostate cancer.

- Preventive strategies that are currently being explored are primarily based on findings from case–control and epidemiological studies.

- Prospective, controlled, clinical trials are needed.

5α-Reductase inhibitors

- Androgens are required for normal prostate development and prostate carcinogenesis.

- ♂ with inherited deficiency of type 2 5α-reductase do not develop benign prostatic hyperplasia (BPH) or prostate cancer.

- 5α-Reductase inhibits the conversion of testosterone to dihydrotestosterone (DHT).

- 5α-Reductase reduces the level of DHT, the most potent androgen in the prostate.

- Type 2 5α-reductase: the predominant isoform in normal prostate and BPH tissue.

- Type 1 5α-reductase: present in BPH tissue and some prostate cancers.

- Approved by the US Food and Drug Administration for the treatment of BPH.

- Finasteride inhibits type 2 isoenzyme, and dutasteride is a type 1 and 2 isoenzyme 5α-reductase inhibitor.

- **Prostate Cancer Prevention Trial (PCPT)**
  [Thompson IM, *N Engl J Med* **349**: 215–224, 2003]
  - First, large-scale, chemoprevention trial in prostate cancer.
  - Double-blind, randomized, multicenter, placebo-controlled, phase III trial.
  - 18,882 ♂ aged > 55 years, prostate-specific antigen (PSA) ≤ 3.0 ng/ml and normal digital rectal examination (DRE), recruited from 1993 to 1996.
  - Primary endpoint: the prevalence of prostate cancer during the 7 years of study, as diagnosed by either for-cause biopsies or by end-of-study biopsy.
  - DESIGN:
    - Randomized to finasteride 5 mg/day or placebo for 7 years.
    - Follow-up: annual DRE and PSA test.
    - Prostate biopsy if the annual PSA level (adjusted for the effect of finasteride) > 4.0 ng/ml or if the DRE was abnormal.
    - At 7 years all ♂ without prostate cancer were offered an end-of-study prostate biopsy.
    - PSA measurements for ♂ in the finasteride group were adjusted to ensure that both groups had an approximately equal recommendation rate for prostate biopsy.
  - RESULTS:
    - 803 of the 4,368 ♂ in the finasteride group (18.4%) and 1,147 of the 4,692 ♂ in the placebo group (24.4%) developed biopsy-proven prostate cancer.
    - There was a 24.8% relative risk (RR) reduction in the prevalence of prostate cancer in the finasteride group (RR = 0.75; 95% confidence interval (CI), 18.6–30.6; $p < 0.001$).
    - Absolute risk reduction 6%; number needed to treat 16.
    - Subgroup analysis: Similar risk reductions were noted among all pre-specified subgroups, which included age, race, family history of prostate cancer, and PSA level at randomization.
    - Risk reduction was seen both in ♂ diagnosed for-cause during the study period or by the end-of-study biopsy.

- The prevalence of Gleason grade 7–10 tumors was higher in the finasteride group compared with the placebo group: 6.4% vs 5.1% (RR = 1.27; 95% CI, 1.07–1.50; p = 0.005).
- Gleason scores for prostate cancers detected:

Gleason score	No. (%) of patients	
	Finasteride group	Placebo group
2–5	89 (11.7%)	173 (16.1%)
6	388 (51.3%)	658 (61.6%)
7–10	280 (37.0%)	237 (22.2%)
All cancers	803 (18.4%)	1147 (24.4%)
All ♂ evaluated	4368	4692
Biopsy for-cause	1639	1934
Positive for cancer	435	571
End-of-study biopsy	3652	3820
Positive for cancer	368	576

- Overall survival and prostate-cancer-specific mortality were not different in the two groups.
- SIDE-EFFECTS:
  - Sexual side-effects were more common among patients who received finasteride: reduced volume of ejaculate, erectile dysfunction, loss of libido, and gynecomastia (p < 0.001 for all comparisons).
  - Urinary symptoms were more common with placebo.

Gleason score	No. (%) of patients	
	Finasteride group	Placebo group
Sexual or endocrine effects		
Reduced ejaculate volume	5690 (60.4%)	4473 (47.3%)
Erectile dysfunction	6349 (67.4%)	5816 (61.5%)
Loss of libido	6163 (65.4%)	5635 (59.6%)
Gynecomastia	426 (4.5%)	261 (2.8%)
Breast cancer	1 (< 0.1%)	1 (< 0.1%)
Genitourinary effects		
BPH	488 (5.2%)	823 (8.7%)
Urinary urgency or frequency	1214 (12.9%)	1474 (15.6%)
Urinary incontinence	183 (1.9%)	208 (2.2%)
Urinary retention	398 (4.2%)	597 (6.3%)

Transurethral resection of the prostate	96 (1.0%)	180 (1.9%)
Prostatitis	418 (4.4%)	576 (6.1%)
Urinary tract infection	90 (1.0%)	126 (1.3%)

- DISCUSSION:
  [Scardino PT, *N Engl J Med* **349**: 297–299, 2003]
  [Parnes HL, *J Clin Oncol* **23**: 368–377, 2005]
  [Mellon JK, *Eur J Cancer* **41**: 2016–2022, 2005]
  [Klein EA, *J Clin Oncol* **23**: 7460–7466, 2005]
  - Long-term follow-up and further laboratory research is needed to determine the reason for the association between finasteride and higher grade prostate cancer.
  - There are several hypotheses:
    - Grading bias: histologic changes that mimic high-grade disease.
    - Finasteride induces high-grade tumors by reducing the level of intraprostatic DHT.
    - Finasteride resulted in the selection of the high-grade tumors by selectively inhibiting low-grade tumors.
  - The clinical significance of cancers found in the end-of-study biopsies is unknown.
  - No overall or cancer-specific survival differences were observed.

Selenium

- Selenium is an essential trace element and is involved in the processes that protect against DNA damage from reactive oxygen species.

- Selenium inhibits tumorigenesis in vivo by a number of potential mechanisms, such as blocking cell proliferation, induction of apoptosis, and cell-cycle arrest.

- **The Netherlands Cohort Study (NLCS)**
  [Van Den Brandt PA, *Cancer Epidemiol Biomarker Prev* **12**: 866–871, 2003]
  - Case cohort study.
  - 58,279 ♂ aged 55–69 years at entry.
  - Participants completed a mailed questionnaire on risk factors for cancer, and provided toenail clippings for selenium tissue quantification.

- RESULTS:
  - Follow-up → 6.3 years from 1986 to 1992.
  - 540 incident prostate carcinoma cases.
  - 1,211 subcohort members with complete toenail selenium data were available for analyses.
  - Multivariate survival analysis showed an inverse association between baseline toenail selenium level and prostate cancer risk.
  - Incident rate ratios in increasing selenium quintiles were 1.00, 1.05, 0.69, 0.75, and 0.69 with RR = 0.69 comparing the highest and lowest quintiles (95% CI, 0.48–0.99; p trend < 0.008).

- **The Nutritional Prevention of Cancer (NPC) Trial**
  [Duffielo-Lillico AJ, *Br J Urol Int* **91**: 608–612, 2003]
  - Designed to evaluate the effect of selenium supplementation on the incidence of non-melanoma skin cancer (not prostate cancer).
  - Randomized, double-blind, placebo-controlled study.
  - 1,312 participants from the eastern USA, with a prior history of skin cancer.
  - No specific eligibility criteria related to prostate cancer.
  - Randomized:
    - Group I: 200 µg/day of selenium as selenized yeast.
    - Group II: placebo.
  - Endpoints:
    - Primary: the incidence of non-melanoma skin cancer.
    - Secondary: the incidence of other cancers, including lung, prostate, and colorectal cancer, and total cancer mortality.
  - RESULTS:
    - Mean follow-up → 7.45 years.
    - Marked reduction in incidence of prostate cancer with selenium supplementation (RR = 0.51; 95% CI, 0.29–0.87).
    - Subgroup analysis:
      - The protective effect was confined to those with PSA ≤ 4 ng/ml (RR = 0.35; 95% CI, 0.13–0.87) and with the lowest two tertiles (< 123.2 ng/ml) of baseline plasma selenium concentrations.

Vitamin E (α-tocopherol)

- Vitamin E is a major lipid-soluble antioxidant, a chain-breaking, free-radical scavenger, and inhibits lipid peroxidation.
- α-Tocopherol is the most active form of vitamin E.

- Large prospective, controlled trials have not yet produced consistent evidence of the efficacy of vitamin E in preventing cancer.

- **Alpha-Tocopherol, Beta-Carotene Cancer Prevention (ATBC) Trial**
  [Heinonen O, *N Engl J Med* **330**: 1029–1035, 1994]
  [Voltamo J, *JAMA* **290**: 476–485, 2003]
  [Heinonen OP, *J Natl Cancer Inst* **90**: 440–446, 1998]
  - Randomized, double-blind, placebo-controlled, primary prevention trial to determine whether supplements of α-tocopherol or β-carotene would reduce the incidence of lung cancer (not prostate cancer).
  - 29,133 ♂ smokers from south-west Finland aged 50–69 years.
  - Randomized to one of four regimens:
    - Group I: α-tocopherol 50 mg/day.
    - Group II: β-carotene 20 mg/day.
    - Group III: α-tocopherol 50 mg/day + β-carotene 20 mg/day.
    - Group IV: placebo.
  - End points:
    - Primary: lung cancer incidence and mortality.
    - Secondary: incidence of other cancers, including prostate cancer.
  - Median follow-up → 6.1 years.
  - RESULTS:
    - 246 incident cases of prostate cancer.
    - 43 were in the α-tocopherol alone group.
    - 56 were in the α-tocopherol + β-carotene group.
    - 80 were in the β-carotene group.
    - 67 were in the placebo group.
    - 32% ↓ in prostate cancer incidence (95% CI, 12–47; $p = 0.0022$) among ♂ receiving α-tocopherol compared with those not receiving it.
    - 41% lower mortality from the prostate cancer in the α-tocopherol group (95% CI, 1–65).
    - Beneficial effects disappeared after discontinuation of the supplement during a 6-year post-intervention follow-up, possibly suggesting that these agents affect the risk of cancer in real time.

- **Beta-Carotene and Retinol Efficacy (CARET) Trial**
  [Goodman GE, *Cancer Epidemiol Biomarker Prev* **12**: 518–526, 2003]
  - A prospective, nested, case–control study to examine any potential association between serum carotenoids, retinoids, and tocopherols on prostate cancer incidence.
  - Randomized, double blind, placebo-controlled lung cancer prevention trial.

- 18,314 patients.
  - 4,060 ♂ asbestos workers.
  - 14,254 ♂ and ♀ (44%) heavy smokers.
- Randomized:
  - Group I: β-carotene 30 mg/day.
  - Group II: retinol 25,000 IU/day.
- RESULTS:
  - High serum levels of α-tocopherol were associated with a lower risk of prostate cancer with a protective odds ratio (OR) of 0.59 (95% CI, 0.34–1.04; p trend = 0.04) for the fourth quartile compared with the first quartile.
  - Risk of prostate cancer by quartile of micronutrient distribution:

	Quartile				
	First	Second	Third	Fourth	p trend
α-Tocopherol	1	0.72	0.61	0.59	0.04

- **The Supplementation of Vitamins and Mineral Antioxidants (SU.VI.MAX) Trial**
  [Mcyer F, *Int J Cancer* **116**: 182–186, 2005]
  [Hercberg S, *Arch Intern Med* **164**: 2335–2342, 2004]
  - Large, population-based, randomized, double-blind, placebo-controlled trial designed to assess whether daily consumption of nutritional doses of antioxidant vitamins and minerals for 8 years could reduce the incidence of cancer and ischemic heart disease.
  - 13,017 volunteers; 7,876 ♀ aged 35–60 years and 5,141 ♂ aged 45–60 years.
  - Randomized:
    - Group I: one capsule containing combination of vitamin C 120 mg, α-tocopherol 30 mg, β-carotene 6 mg, selenium 100 μg, and zinc 20 mg.
    - Group II: placebo.
  - Median follow-up:
    - Supplementation group → 9.0 years.
    - Placebo arm → 8.8 years.
  - RESULTS:
    - An adjunct study was conducted to assess whether the supplements could ↓ the occurrence of prostate cancer in 3,161 ♂.
    - 103 new cases of prostate cancer with 49/2,522 ♂ in the supplement group and 54/2,512 ♂ in the placebo group (hazard ratio (HR) = 0.88; 95% CI, 0.60–1.29).

- With baseline PSA < 3 ng/ml: significant reduction in the rate of prostate cancer with supplementation (HR = 0.52; 95% CI, 0.29–0.92; p = 0.009).
- With PSA ≥ 3 ng/ml: HR = 1.54 (95% CI, 0.87–2.72).

Selective estrogen receptor modulators

- Rationale: non-steroidal compounds with weak estrogen- and cancer-suppressing activity.

- Toremifene, a chlorinated derivative of tamoxifen.

- Phase III, placebo-controlled, randomized, industry-sponsored clinical trial.
    - ♂ with high-grade prostatic intraepithelial neoplasia (HGPIN) on biopsy, PSA ≤ 10 ng/ml.
    - Randomized:
        - Group I: toremifene citrate 20 mg/day for 18 months.
        - Group II: placebo
    - Prostate biopsies planned at 12 and 18 months.

Soy

- Active agent: major source of isoflavones, mainly in the form of genistein.

- Has estrogen-like activity because of the structural similarity to human estrogens, and is known to inhibit 5α-reductase.

- Isoflavones have also been shown to inhibit benign and malignant prostatic epithelial growth, down-regulate androgen-regulated genes, and reduce tumor growth in some animal models.

- Ongoing trials:
    - NCI: phase II, randomized, double-blind, placebo-controlled trial.
        - Dietary soy protein supplement for 12 months in patients with elevated PSA levels (5–10 ng/ml) and a negative biopsy for prostate cancer.
    - NCI of Canada PRP-1: 310 ♂ with HGPIN.
        - Randomized to placebo or a soy-based powder containing supplemental vitamin E and selenium.
        - Biopsy at 6, 12, 24, and 36 months.
        - Anticipated results in late 2007.

Lycopene

[Kucuk O, *Cancer Epidemiol Biomarker Prev* **10**: 861–868, 2001]
[Chen L, *J Natl Cancer Inst* **93**: 1872–1879, 2001]
[Giovannucci E, *J Nutr* 135: 2030S–2031S, 2005]

- A red-orange carotenoid found primarily in tomatoes and tomato-derived products, and the predominant carotenoid in human plasma.

- It is known to have potent antioxidant activity, and inhibits the growth of benign and malignant prostatic epithelial cells in vitro.

- Only small clinical trials have examined the effect of lycopene on known prostate cancer, and the results from epidemiological studies are controversial.

- Ongoing, phase I trial sponsored by the National Cancer Institute.

Major ongoing trials

- Reduction by Dutasteride of Prostate Cancer Events (REDUCE) Trial
  [Andriole G, *J Urol* **172**: 1314–1317, 2004]
  [Gomella L, *Curr Opin Urol* **15**: 29–32, 2005]
  - Ongoing trial.
  - Randomized, double-blind, placebo-controlled trial currently underway in the USA and Europe.
  - Involving 650 centers, the trial has completed an accrual of 8,000 ♂.
  - Target population:
    - ♂ at ↑ risk of prostate cancer but with no evidence of disease at study entry.
    - Age 50–75 years.
    - PSA 2.5–10 ng/ml for ♂ aged 50–60 years or ≥ 3–10 ng/ml for ♂ aged > 60 years.
    - Negative 6–12 core biopsy for both cancer and HGPIN or atypical acinar proliferation within 6 months prior to enrolment.
  - Primary end point → the rate of biopsy-proven prostate cancer.
  - Randomized:
    - Group I: dutasteride 0.5 mg/day for 4 years.
    - Group II: placebo.
  - Follow-up: PSA level measured every 6 months with repeat 10-core biopsy at years 2 and 4.

- **The Selenium and Vitamin E Cancer Prevention (SELECT) Trial**
  [Klein EA, *Ann NY Acad Sci* **1031**: 234–241, 2004]

- Phase III, randomized, double-blind, prospective trial to determine whether selenium and/or vitamin E can ↓ the risk of prostate cancer among healthy ♂.
- Eligibility criteria:
  - Age ≥ 50 years for African Americans, ≥ 55 years for Caucasians.
  - DRE not indicating cancer.
  - PSA ≤ 4.0 ng/ml.
- Randomized:
  - Group I: L-selenomethionine 200 μg.
  - Group II: 400 mg of racemic α-tocopheryl supplements.
  - Group III: placebo.
  - Group IV: L-selenomethionine 200 μg + 400 mg of racemic α-tocopheryl supplements.
- Study duration → 7–12 years.
- Follow-up: annual DRE and PSA, and routine clinical diagnostic work-up as indicated.
- Endpoints:
  - Primary: clinical incidence of prostate cancer.
  - Secondary: prostate-cancer-free survival, all-cause mortality, and incidence of and mortality from other cancers and disease.
- Target accrual of 32,400 ♂ reached in 2004.
  - Initial data analysis: 2006.
  - Final results: 2013.

5

Prostate-specific antigen and digital rectal examination screening for prostate cancer

Introduction

[Labric F, *Prostate* **38**: 83, 1999]
[Hankey BF, *J Natl Cancer Inst* **91**: 1017, 1999]
[Etzioni R, *J Natl Cancer Inst* **94**: 981, 2002]
[Rietbergen JB, *Acta Oncol* **37**: 515, 1998]

- There is no consensus on whether screening for prostate cancer is beneficial or not.

- There is no definite evidence to demonstrate a significant $\downarrow$ in disease mortality due to screening and early detection of prostate cancer.

- Retrospective studies suggest significant stage migration, with resultant improved survival advantage.

- Digital rectal examination (DRE) and prostate-specific antigen (PSA) are widely used as initial screening tools for prostate cancer detection.

Digital rectal examination

[Carvalhal GF, *J Urol* **161**: 835, 1999]
[Schroder FH, *J Natl Cancer Inst* **90**: 1817, 1998]
[Catalona WJ, *J Urol* **151**: 1283, 1994]

- DRE (Fig. 5.1) is an integral part of the clinical evaluation of a patient with suspected prostate cancer.

- Abnormal DRE is the second most common finding, after PSA, which initiates further studies towards the diagnosis of prostate cancer.

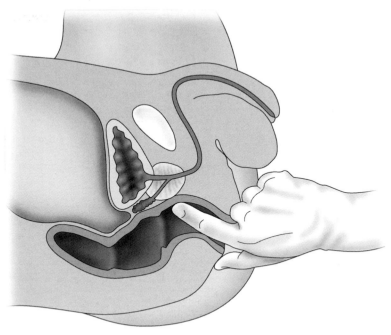

Fig. 5.1 Digital rectal examination of the prostate.

- Interobserver and intraobserver variation is very high, resulting in low reproducibility of the findings.
- A formal DRE can be done in the erect position or the lateral decubitus position.
  - The size, surface, and consistency of the prostate should be noted.
- Abnormal DRE findings in patients with prostate cancer include:
  - A nodule.
  - Asymmetry.
  - Hard mass.
- The size of the prostate does <u>not</u> correlate with the incidence of prostate cancer.

Is DRE a good diagnostic and screening tool?

- Most prostate cancer patients in the modern era do not have any abnormality on DRE.
- Most patients with an abnormal DRE are asymptomatic.

- Although an abnormal DRE has a high positive predictive value, only a small number of patients are diagnosed solely on the basis of an abnormal DRE.

- DRE has low sensitivity and specificity.

- DRE is associated with significant understaging of disease.

- DRE is not recommended as a sole diagnostic or screening tool for prostate cancer.

Transrectal ultrasonography of the prostate

[Mettlin C, CA Cancer J Clin **47**: 265, 1997]
[Flanigan RC, J Urol **152**: 1506, 1994]
[Goto Y, Int J Urol **5**: 337, 1998]
[Narayan P, Urology **46**: 205, 1995]

- Transrectal ultrasonography (TRUS) is usually used as an adjunct tool when undertaking a biopsy of the prostate and when making a volume measurement of the prostate for brachytherapy.

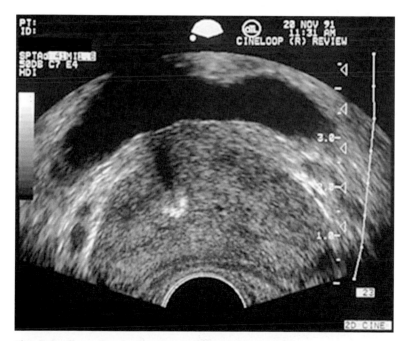

Fig. 5.2 Transrectal ultrasound scan of the prostate.

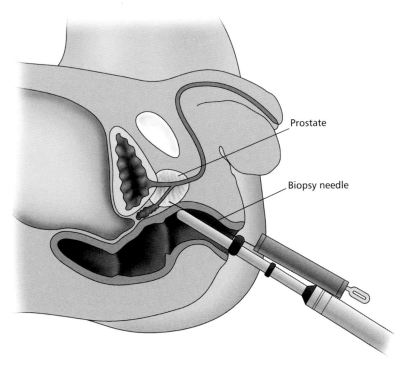

Fig. 5.3 Transrectal ultrasound of the prostate.

- The most common TRUS finding in prostate cancer is a hypoechoic lesion (Figs 5.2 and 5.3).

- TRUS <u>cannot</u> identify small lesions (< 0.5 cm) and prostate cancer may be isoechoic.

- TRUS has low positive predictive value and specificity.

- DRE combined with PSA level has a better predictive value than the combination of DRE and TRUS (Table 5.1).

- TRUS is expensive.

- Hence TRUS is not routinely used as an initial screening tool.

Prostate-specific antigen

[Polascik TJ, *J Urol* **162**: 293, 1999]
[Konety BR, *J Urol* **174**: 1785, 2005]

Table 5.1 The American Cancer Society National Prostate Cancer Detection Project report on different screening tools for prostate cancer detection

Diagnostic tool	Positive predictive value
DRE	8%
TRUS	6%
DRE + PSA	32%
DRE + TRUS	13%
PSA + TRUS	32%
DRE + PSA + TRUS	51.5%

[Loeb S, *J Urol* **175**: 902, 2006]
[Stamey TA, *J Urol* **172**: 1297, 2004]

- PSA is a 33 kDa, androgen-regulated, serine protease that is primarily produced by the prostate epithelium and epithelial lining of the periurethral glands.

- The standard PSA reference range is 0.0–4.0 ng/ml.

- The half-life of PSA is 2.2–3.2 days.

- Although not cancer specific, estimation of organ-specific serum PSA remains the most widely used tumor marker for prostate cancer.

- Serum PSA levels can be temporarily altered by various pharmacological therapies, prostatic disease, and urological interventions.

- Annual PSA screening for prostate cancer for all ♂ ≥ 50 years old is recommended by the American Urological Association and the American Cancer Society.

- Screening should start at age 40 years for ♂ with a family history of prostate cancer or for ♂ of African American descent.

- Since the introduction of PSA testing into clinical practice in late 1980s, the incidence of localized prostate cancer initially markedly ↑, and then showed signs of a major ↓ in the late 1990s, while regional and metastatic prostate cancers have declined continuously.

- PSA testing with DRE improves the detection of prostate cancer and has ↑ the lead time for diagnosis.

- With widespread screening, the prevalence of latent prostate cancer has ↓ three-fold.

- Recent studies showed that the majority (~ 90%) of screening-detected cancers met the pathological criteria for significant cancer.

Age-specific PSA

[Oesterling JE, JAMA **270**: 860, 1993]
[Morgan TO, N Engl J Med **335**: 304, 1996]
[Nadler RB, J Urol **174**: 2154, 2005]

- The standard PSA reference range (0.0–4.0 ng/ml) does not compensate for age and volume changes due to benign prostatic hyperplasia (BPH).

- Age-specific reference ranges (Table 5.2) have the potential to make the serum PSA level more specific in older ♂, thus avoiding unnecessary biopsies, and more sensitive in younger ♂ (age < 60 years), thus diagnosing more localized disease.

- Although widely accepted, discretion should be used when using these values for high-risk groups.

- Recent evidence suggests that a lower PSA cut-off level of 2.5 ng/ml could be considered, irrespective of age, in ♂ who would be candidates for definitive treatment.

Table 5.2 Age-specific PSA reference ranges

Age (years)	Normal PSA range (ng/ml)	
	Black men	White men
40–49	0–2.0	0–2.5
50–59	0–4.0	0–3.5
60–69	0–4.5	0–4.5
70–79	0–5.5	0–6.5

PSA density

[Benson MC, *J Urol* **147**: 817, 1992]
[Catalona WJ, *J Urol* **152**: 2031, 1994]
[Kalish J, *Urology* **43**: 601, 1994]
[Djavan B, *J Urol* **160**: 411, 1998]
[Jain S, *Postgrad Med J* **78**: 646, 2002]

- The theory that prostate cancer releases more PSA per volume unit than BPH led to the concept of PSA density.

- PSA density is defined as the total serum PSA level (ng/ml) divided by the TRUS-determined prostate volume (cm^3).

- The ability of serum PSA to differentiate cancer from BPH is particularly poor in the intermediate range (4–10 ng/ml) with a normal DRE.

- The PSA density could distinguish cancer from BPH.
  - A threshold value of 0.15 has been suggested as a discriminatory point for cancer.

- The prostate volume estimated using TRUS is an operator-dependent factor that is a limitation in the PSA density calculation.

- Large multicenter studies have reported that the PSA density has not been an effective tool for assessing the need for prostate biopsy in ♂ with PSA levels in the range 4–10 ng/ml and with a normal DRE.

- Further attempts to improve the specificity of PSA density as a screening tool led to the concept of transition-zone PSA density (PSA/cm^3 of transition-zone volume), which accounts for the proportion of PSA produced by the transition zone.

- Transition-zone PSA remains an investigatory tool.

PSA velocity

[Carter HB, *Cancer Res* **52**: 3323, 1992]
[Smith DS, *J Urol* **152**: 1163, 1994]

- The PSA velocity is defined as the rate of ↑ in serum PSA over time.

- A minimum of three PSA level measurements should be obtained over a 2-year period, or at least 12–18 months apart, to obtain maximum benefit.

- PSA velocity = $\frac{1}{2}(PSA_2 - PSA_1$/$time_1$ in years$) + (PSA_3 - PSA_2$/$time_2$ in years).

- A PSA velocity of 0.75 ng/ml per year is the suggested threshold level for ♂ aged ≤ 70 years with a normal PSA level.

- A threshold level of 0.4 ng/ml per year is more strongly predictive for cancer in ♂ with a PSA level > 4.0 ng/ml.

- Limitations of the PSA velocity is that the PSA level varies significantly (up to 25% in the same individual) over time and different assays.

- The PSA velocity may be useful in monitoring ♂ with a negative initial biopsy.

Free PSA and percentage free PSA

[Catalona WJ, JAMA **279**: 1542, 1998]
[Catalona WJ, *Urology* **56**: 255, 2000]
[Collins GN, *J Urol* **157**: 1744, 1997]
[Khan MA, *J Urol* **170**: 723, 2003]

- PSA that reaches the serum is either free or bound to plasma proteins.
    - α-1-Antichymotrypsin (ACT), α-2-macroglobulin (A2M), and α-1-protease inhibitor (API) are well-known binding proteins for PSA.

- When bound to A2M, PSA is not detectable by standard methods.

- Total PSA (tPSA) = free PSA + ACT PSA + API PSA.

- The probability of prostate cancer is inversely related to the percentage of free PSA (fPSA).

- The challenge is to determine the best threshold level to rule out BPH, while detecting cancer.
    - It appears that 25% may be the optimum level for PSA levels in the range 4.0–10.0 ng/ml.
    - This has been shown to detect 95% of cancers and to eliminate 20% of unnecessary prostate biopsies.
    - In the range 2.5–4.0 ng/ml PSA, a threshold of 27% has been shown to detect ~ 90% of cancers while eliminating 18% of unnecessary biopsies.

- The percentage fPSA is used to increase the sensitivity of cancer detection when the tPSA is normal (≤ 4.0 ng/ml), and to improve the specificity when the tPSA is elevated (4–10 ng/ml).

- Studies have also suggested that the percentage fPSA may predict tumor aggressiveness several years before tPSA.

- The serum fPSA should be assayed within 3 hours of serum collection; serum should be stored at −70°C if not processed within 24 hours.

- At present, percentage fPSA plays an important role in determining whether a patient with a normal DRE and a tPSA in the range 4–10 ng/ml would benefit from biopsy or rebiopsy.

- Pro-PSA, which is a derivative of fPSA, has truncated forms.
  - [–2] pro-PSA, [–4] pro-PSA and full length [–7] pro-PSA.
  - There is evidence that pro-PSA is preferentially associated with prostate cancer.

- The sum of pro-PSA, tPSA, and fPSA improves the specificity of early prostate cancer detection in ♂ with a tPSA in the range 4–10 ng/ml.

- fPSA and the percentage fPSA are altered by all forms of prostatic manipulations.
  - Phlebotomy must precede DRE and other prostatic manipulations in order to avoid misleading results.

Complexed PSA

[Allard WJ, *Clin Chem* **44:** 1216, 1998]
[Brawer MK, *Urology* **52:** 372, 1998]
[Finne P, *J Urol* **164:** 1956, 2000]
[Jung K, *J Urol* **175:** 1275, 2006]
[Horninger W, *Urology* **60:** 31, 2002]
[Oesterling JE, *J Urol* **154:** 1090, 1995]

- Attempts to improve the specificity of PSA testing led to the concept of complexed PSA (cPSA), which is bound to ACT.

- Both the serum concentration and the proportion of complex PSA (ACT) were substantially higher than the tPSA in ♂ with prostate cancer than in ♂ with BPH.

- Another study reported that the proportion of serum PSA API was significantly lower in ♂ with prostate cancer.
  - Incorporation of this finding into the analysis improved the specificity of fPSA and tPSA in the screening of the population with levels in the range 4–10 ng/ml.

- A review of the diagnostic performances of tPSA and cPSA resulted in controversial interpretations.

- Recent studies that employed the discordance analysis characteristics

(DAC) method to assess the predictive value of cPSA showed promising outcomes.
- cPSA showed a 3.6- to 5.5-fold better specificity and avoided 10% of unnecessary biopsies in ♂ with PSA in the range 3–5 ng/ml.

- Larger, prospective, multicenter studies are required to evaluate fully the place of this new investigatory tool.

New serum markers and novel techniques

[Stephan C, *Prostate* **66**: 651, 2006]
[Snow PB, *J Urol* **161** (Suppl 4S): 210, 1999]

- Human kallikrein 2 (hK2).
  - There is high hK2 expression in prostate cancer cells.
  - hK2 expression shows 80% homology with PSA.
  - The hK2/fPSA ratio showed improved specificity.

- Prostate-specific membrane antigen (PSMA).
  - PSMA is highly prostate specific.
  - Detection of PSMA in serum implies the presence of circulating prostate cells.
  - Detection of PSMA is useful in effective differentiation between cancer and BPH when PSA is in the range 4–10 ng/ml.

- Artificial neural networks.
  - Artificial neural networks incorporate age, race, DRE, PSA, and fPSA into a single model.
  - Artificial neural networks are 25–40% more predictive of a positive biopsy than are PSA or fPSA.
  - This helps the physician to counsel the patient regarding prostate biopsy.
  - Artificial neural networks with the novel input factors of MIC-1, MIF, and/or hK11 demonstrated a significant advantage compared with percentage fPSA and tPSA in avoiding unnecessary prostate biopsies.

Prostate cancer: imaging features

Ultrasound: transrectal ultrasonography

[Rummack CM, *Diagnostic Ultrasound*, 3rd edn. Mosby, Edinburgh, 2005]
[Frauscher F, *Ultrasound Q* **18**(2): 135–140, 2002]

- ~ 60–70% of prostate cancers can be detected using transrectal ultrasonography (TRUS) (Fig. 6.1(a)).

- Indications:
  - Abnormal PSA levels.
  - Clinically palpable nodules (digital rectal examination (DRE)).
  - Ultrasound guidance for biopsy procedures.
  - Staging of known prostate cancer.
  - Monitoring of response to treatment.

TRUS imaging features

- Generally <u>hypoechoic</u> (the lesion appears dark relative to the surrounding tissue).
  - Corresponds pathologically to lower grade and better differentiated cancer.

- Differential diagnosis for hypoechoic lesion:
  - Atypical hyperplasia; chronic prostatitis; nodules of benign prostatic hyperplasia, infarcts.

- Less commonly hyperechoic (the lesion appears bright relative to the surrounding tissue).

- Correlates pathologically with a desmoplastic response with a cribriform pattern or comedonecrosis.

- Rarely, isoechoic (the lesion is of the same brightness as the surrounding tissue), and hence impossible to detect.
  - Secondary signs, such as asymmetry or focal bulge, are helpful.
  - This type probably correlates with a diffuse type of cancer.

- Role of color Doppler ultrasonography (non-specific) (Fig. 6.1(b)).
  - There is no ↑ benefit over grayscale ultrasonography, as non-malignant conditions also show ↑ vascularity.

- Positive predictive value:
  - 30–40% if the sole criterion for diagnosis is hypoechogenicity (the lesion appears dark relative to the surrounding tissue) of the lesion.
  - ↑ to 50% when prostate-specific antigen (PSA) level is also ↑.
  - Further ↑ to 60% when associated with palpable abnormality (DRE).
  - ↑ to 70% when both criteria (elevated PSA and palpable nodule on DRE) are utilized.

Computerized tomography

[Haaga JR, Lanzieri CF, *CT and MR Imaging of the Whole Body*, Vol. 2, 4th edn, Mosby, New York, 2003]
[Lee JKT, *Computed Body Tomography with MRI Correlation*, Vol. 2, 4th edn. Lippincott, Williams & Wilkins, Baltimore, OH, 2005]

- Because of low sensitivity for the detection of extracapsular spread in early stage prostate cancer, computerized tomography (CT) is not effective in staging the T_2 or early T_3 stages.

- Indications:
  - To confirm the findings of DRE in bulky and advanced disease.
  - To plan radiation therapy.

- Overall accuracy in detecting extracapsular spread → 58–64%.

CT imaging features

- Irregular enhancement of soft-tissue density tumor with surrounding fat stranding.
  - Many benign inflammatory conditions could produce the same findings.

- Obliteration of fat planes with adjacent structures.

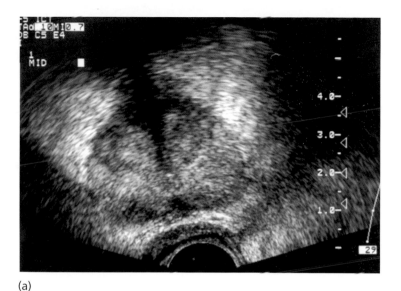

(a)

(b)

Fig. 6.1 (a) TRUS scan of the prostate demonstrates two hypoechoic areas within the right peripheral zone and in the midline, suggestive of prostatic carcinoma. (b) The same area demonstrates hypervascularity in the same area in the Doppler ultrasound image. These areas were proven to represent cancer in subsequent ultrasound-guided biopsies. (Courtesy of Professor Amendola Marco and Assistant Professor Prasanna Kumar, Department of Radiology, University of Miami, FL, USA.)

- Loss of angle between the prostate and the seminal vesicle.

- Detection of lymph node metastasis, accuracy → 67–93%, with a size threshold of 6 mm.
  - Predictable and stepwise involvement: the obturator group, then the common iliac and presacral group of lymph nodes. The para-aortic region is involved in the late stages.

- When evaluating recurrent disease, the pattern of disease presentation is different.
  - Predominantly upper abdominal retroperitoneal disease process is demonstrated.

- Dynamic CT perfusion study of the prostate is claimed to be more sensitive in detecting poorly differentiated cancer with high tumor volume.
  - Results are yet to be validated in large prospective studies.
    [Ives EP, *Clin Prostate Cancer* 4(2):109–112, 2005]

Magnetic resonance imaging and magnetic resonance spectroscopy

[Haaga JR, Lanzieri CF, *CT and MR Imaging of the Whole Body*, Vol. 2, 4th edn. Mosby, New York, 2003].

- T1 and T2 weighted images in the axial, sagital, and coronal planes are obtained. Use of intravenous gadolinium contrast agent is favored.
  - T2 weighted images are the best in depicting the peripheral and central zones, and the prostate cancer.
  - High-resolution images can be obtained using an endorectal coil.

- Sensitivity → 51–89%; specificity → 67–87%.
  - Accuracy is as high as 82–88%.
    [Huch-Boni RA, *Clin Radiol* 50: 593–600, 1995]
    [Bartolozzi C, *Eur Radiol* 6: 339–345, 1996]

- Statistically significant prediction ($p < 0.05$) of early vs late stage was demonstrated in a cohort study.
  [D'Amico AV, *J Clin Oncol* 14: 1770–1777, 1996]

MRI imaging features

- Low signal intensity (the lesion appears dark relative to the surrounding peripheral bright zone) on T2 weighted images (Fig.6.2(a, b)).

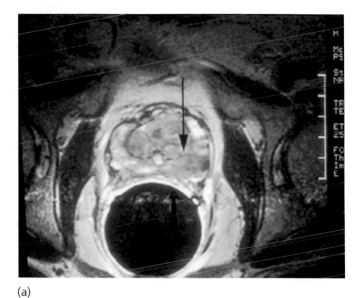

(a)

(b)

Fig. 6.2 MRI scan of the prostate obtained using an endorectal coil.
(a) Axial T2 weighted image showing prostate cancer as a dark signal
area (arrow) within the bright peripheral zone. (b) Coronal T2 weighted
image demonstrating the same tumor in the left peripheral zone.
(Courtesy of Professor Amendola Marco and Assistant Professor
Prasanna Kumar, Department of Radiology, University of Miami, FL, USA.)

- Obliteration of the rectoprostatic angle is one of the signs of prostatic extension.
- Asymmetry of the neurovascular bundles because of macroscopic perineural invasion.
  – One common site → posterolateral edge of the prostate (Fig. 6.3).
- Surrounding fat plane obliteration.
- Irregular bulging of the prostatic capsule.
- Asymmetry of the seminal vesicles with low signal intensities on T2 weighted images.
  – Obliteration of the fat plane between the prostate and the seminal vesicles suggests a direct extension of metastatic spread to the seminal vesicles (Figs 6.4(a, b)).
- Reasons for false-negative results:
  – Rare, central gland tumor.
  – Tumors surrounded by hemorrhage (post-biopsy) or inflammatory processes.
  – Tumors infiltrating the stroma of the peripheral zone.

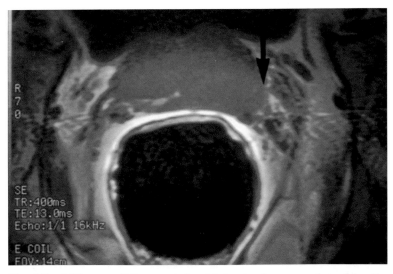

Fig. 6.3 MRI scan of the prostate obtained using an endorectal coil. Axial T1 weighted image demonstrating tumor invading the left neurovascular bundle. (Courtesy of Professor Amendola Marco and Assistant Professor Prasanna Kumar, Department of Radiology, University of Miami, FL, USA.)

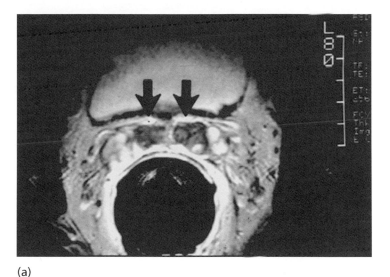

(a)

(b)

Fig. 6.4 MRI scan of the prostate obtained using an endorectal coil.
(a) Axial T2 weighted image displaying a dark signal in both seminal
vesicles, consistent with tumor extensions from prostate cancer.
(b) Coronal T2 weighted image displaying dark signal in both seminal
vesicles, consistent with tumor extensions from prostate cancer
(arrows). (Courtesy of Professor Amendola Marco and Assistant
Professor Prasanna Kumar, Department of Radiology, University of
Miami, FL, USA.)

Magnetic resonance spectroscopy

[Coakley FV, *J Urol* **170**: S69–S76, 2003]

- Magnetic resonance spectroscopy (MRS) (Fig. 6.5(a, b)) provides a more comprehensive metabolic and anatomic evaluation.

- Sensitivity → 68–73% and specificity → 70–80%.

- **It is helpful in differentiating prostate cancer from post-biopsy hemorrhage and other processes**.

- Higher choline levels and lower citrate levels relative to normal tissue have been demonstrated to correlate well with statistically significant cancer aggressiveness and Gleason score.

- The tumor volume estimate, which is a good predictor of extracapsular spread of the tumor, can also be demonstrated using MRS.

- Residual or recurrent cancer can also be detected.

Nuclear medicine studies

[Thrall J, *Nuclear Medicine: The Requisites*, 2nd edn, Mosby, New York, 2001]

- Indium-111 ProstaScint.
  - ProstaScint is used in conjunction with CT scans.
  - Dose: indium-111 ProstaScint 5 mci i.v.
  - ProstaScint requires a single photon emission computerized tomography (SPECT) gamma camera.
  - Images are obtained after 30 minutes, and delayed images of the abdomen and pelvis are obtained after 3–5 days.

- Indications:
  - Biopsy-proven prostate cancer that is clinically staged early and is localized, but where there is high risk of pelvic lymph node metastasis.
  - Post-prostatectomy patients with rising PSA levels.

- Accuracy: in a multicenter trial of 152 patients with a tissue diagnosis of prostate cancer ProstaScint correctly identified 40 of 64 ♂.

- Sensitivity → 62% and specificity → 72%.

Nuclear medicine imaging features:

- An abnormal scan shows as ↑ uptake in the prostate fossa, and its draining lymph nodes.

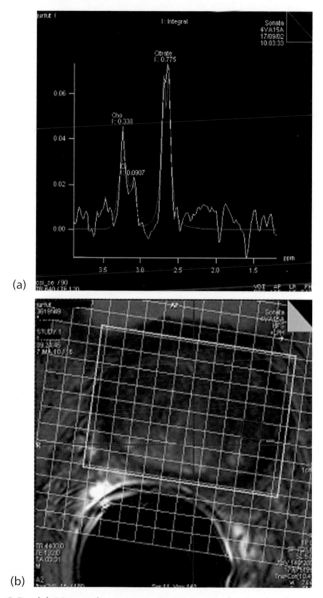

Fig. 6.5 (a) Magnetic resonance spectrum obtained using an endorectal coil and (b) MRS maps, demonstrating increased levels of choline and lower levels of citrate than seen in normal prostate, which are characteristic of prostate cancer. (Courtesy of Professor Amendola Marco and Assistant Professor Prasanna Kumar, Department of Radiology, University of Miami, FL, USA.)

- Images may be obtained utilizing a single isotope (indium-111) on the same day and at 3–5 days.

- Or at 3–5 days after injecting the patient with dual isotopes (technetium-99m and indium-111) for SPECT.

- Interpretation requires specific training, as normal bowel and bladder clearance can cause difficulty in interpretation.

7

Evaluation of abnormal digital rectal examination or elevated prostate-specific antigen

Digital rectal examination

- The prostate gland contains several histologically distinct zones. [McNeal JE, *Am J Surg Pathol* **12**: 619–633, 1988]
    - The majority of prostate cancers occur within the peripheral zone, which is palpable during the digital rectal examination (DRE).
    - ~ 15–25% of tumors occur within the transition zone, which is the region that gives rise to the adenomatous growth characteristic of benign prostatic hyperplasia (BPH).

- <u>DRE of the prostate.</u>
    - The size, shape, and position of the prostate are noted.
    - The median raphe is palpated, and the gloved finger is swept from one side of the gland to the other, examining the prostate from its base to apex.
    - The normal prostate gland is smooth, soft, and homogeneous on DRE, which is performed either in the lateral decubitus position or with the patient standing up and bending forward.
    - Abnormal regions palpated on DRE are characterized as either nodules or areas of induration.
        - They should be described as focal or diffuse, well circumscribed or irregular, within the prostate or extending outside of the prostate, mobile or fixed, tender or non-tender, and whether there is fluctuation.
        - Tenderness or fluctuation is more suggestive of inflammatory or infectious etiologies.

- The differential diagnosis for a prostatic nodule includes:
  - Neoplastic.
    - Adenocarcinoma.
    - Less common tumors, such as transitional cell carcinoma, sarcoma, small-cell carcinoma, and lymphoma, usually present as diffuse firmness or induration, and not as a discrete nodule.
  - Non-neoplastic.
    - Prostatic calculi/concretions.
    - Post-surgical changes.
    - Granulomatous prostatitis.
    - BPH.

Prostate-specific antigen

- Prostate-specific antigen (PSA) is a serine protease with both chymotrypsin- and trypsin-like activity.
  - It is almost exclusively produced by the epithelial acini of the prostate gland, as well as the epithelial cells within the periurethral glands.
  - Its function is not entirely known, but it may play a role in liquefaction of the seminal fluid.

- PSA exists as both protein-bound and free fractions in the serum.
  - The bound fraction of PSA refers to the majority of serum PSA, which is covalently bound to α-1-antichymotrypsin and α-2-macroglobulin.

- Serum PSA that is not bound to serum proteins is present in much smaller quantities within the blood stream.
  - Measurement of the percentage free PSA has been found to improve the specificity of the PSA test in screening for prostate cancer (see below).

- Measurement of the serum PSA in screened populations has confirmed that 85–92% of ♂ have PSA values of ≤ 4.0 ng/ml.
  [Catalona WJ, JAMA **270**: 948–954, 1993]
  [Brawer MK, J Urol **147**: 841–845, 1992]
  [Mettlin CC, Cancer **67**: 2949–2958, 1991]

- ~ 25% of patients with serum PSA values in the range 4–10 ng/ml and a normal DRE will have prostate cancer.
  [Crawford ED, Prostate **38**: 296–302,1999]

- This is similar to the percentage of ♂ having prostate cancer who have PSA values in the range 2.5–4 ng/ml.
  [Catalona WJ, JAMA **277**: 1452–1455, 1997]
  [Smith DS, J Urol **160**: 1734–1738, 1998]

- An ↑ PSA is not specific to prostate cancer. Other causes of an ↑ PSA include:
  - Infection (bladder, seminal vesical, prostate, or urethra).
  - Acute or chronic bacterial prostatitis.
  - Following prostatic manipulation (surgical, biopsy, or trauma). Routine prostate examination is not thought to cause the PSA ↑.
  - Prostatic infarction.
  - Following cardiac bypass.

- Efforts to ↑ the sensitivity and specificity of the serum PSA examination in identifying ♂ with prostate cancer have included the following:
  - **Age-adjusted PSA levels.**
    [Oesterling JE, JAMA **270**(7): 860–864, 1993]

Age (years)	Age-specific reference range (ng/ml)
40–49	0.0–2.5
50–59	0.0–3.5
60–69	0.0–4.5
70–79	0.0–6.5

  - **Race-adjusted PSA levels.**
    [Morgan TO, N Engl J Med **335**: 304–310, 1996]

Age (years)	PSA range (ng/ml)	
	White men	Black men
40–49	0–2.5	0–2.0
50–59	0–3.5	0–4.0
60–69	0–3.5	0–4.5
70–79	0–3.5	0–5.5

  - **PSA velocity.**
    [Carter HB, JAMA **267**: 2215–2220, 1992]
    - Refers to the rate of rise in the serum PSA per year.
    - In this longitudinal study, a PSA velocity of 0.75 ng/ml per year showed a greater likelihood of being associated with carcinoma of the prostate.

Percentage free and total PSA

- Used to enhance the specificity of the PSA indicating prostate cancer.

- The free PSA/total PSA ratio significantly enhanced the specificity of the PSA values in the range 4.0–10.0 ng/ml.
  [Catalona WJ, JAMA **279**(19): 1542–1547, 1998]

- Based on this prospective, multicenter trial, patients with a normal DRE and serum PSA levels in the range 4.1–10 ng/ml have a probability of prostate cancer of:

Percent free PSA	Probability of cancer (%)
0–10	56
10–15	28
15–20	20
20–25	16
> 25	8

- In a prospective, multicenter trial, complexed PSA alone offered improved specificity over the total PSA.
  - Free PSA and the percentage free PSA offered no additional benefit in terms of distinguishing between benign and malignant disease.
    [Partin AW, J Urol **170**: 1787–1791, 2003]

- The free PSA/total PSA ratio improves the specificity in high-risk patients with a total PSA level in the range 2.0–4.0 ng/ml.
  - High-risk patients with a PSA level in the range 2.0–4 ng/ml and a percentage free PSA > 27% had → 52% probability of prostate cancer on prostate biopsy.
    [Uzzo RG, Urology **61**: 754–759, 2003]

Prostate biopsy

- The indications for prostate biopsy traditionally involve either ↑ serum PSA or an abnormal DRE.
  - Additional risk factors, such as age, family history, and race, should also be taken into account in deciding whether a prostate biopsy is performed.

- The decision to perform a prostate biopsy is an individual one between the physician and the patient.
  - Risks and benefits, including the risks of identifying a clinically

insignificant cancer, should be discussed with the patient who is facing the decision of whether to undergo a prostate biopsy.

- For ♂ who have a solitary PSA ↑, confirmation of the abnormal PSA result should be performed prior to biopsy.
  [Eastham JA, JAMA **289**(20): 2695–2700, 2003]

Prostate biopsy technique

- There is no uniformly accepted prostate biopsy protocol.
  - Two studies have shown widely varying patterns of antibiotic administration, use of a preoperative enema, utilization of anesthesia, and the number of biopsy cores taken.
    [Davis M, *J Urol* **167**: 566–570, 2002]
    [Patel HR, *Int J Clin Pract* **57**(9): 773–774, 2003]

- Antibiotic administration.
  - Fluoroquinolones are used as antibiotic prophylaxis for prostate biopsies.
  - There is some variability in the timing of antibiotics.
  - The antibiotic may be started 1 day prior to the procedure, while others administer it just prior to the procedure itself.
  - Continuation of antibiotics for > 24 hours after the biopsy has no sound scientific basis.
  - Guidelines for antibiotic prophylaxis in patients who are at risk of bacterial endocarditis (i.e. artificial heart valve) should be followed.

- Preoperative enema.
  - There are few data supporting the view that a preoperative enema reduces the risk of bacteremia or infectious complications in patients undergoing prostate biopsy.
  - In a retrospective series of 4,439 biopsies, the symptomatic infection rate using ciprofloxacin and no preoperative enema was 0.1%.
    [Sieber PR, *J Urol* **157**: 2199, 1997]
  - Given these data, it would be hard to perform a study with sufficient power to refute the view that a preoperative enema could ↓ the risk of infectious complications.

Prostate analgesia

- [Nash PA, *J Urol* **155**(2): 607–609, 1996]
  - Described the utility of a periprostatic nerve block in patients undergoing prostate biopsy.

- – In this study, unilateral anesthesia was provided to the prostate by infiltrating 1% lidocaine 5 ml into the junction between the prostate and the seminal vesicle.
- – Patients served as their own controls, indicating a ↓ in pain associated with the biopsy of the anesthetized side.

- [Soloway M, *J Urol* **163**: 172–173, 2000]
  [Alavi AS, *J Urol* **166**(4): 1343–1345, 2001]
  [Stirling BN, *Urology* **60**(1): 89–92, 2002]
  [von Knowblock R, *Eur Urol* **41**(5): 508–514, 2002]
  - – Several randomized trials have confirmed its superiority to administering intrarectal lidocaine gel.
  - – 5–10 ml of a 1% xylocaine solution (without epinephrine) is injected via a 70-inch, 22-gauge spinal needle, which is inserted through the transrectal ultrasound probe.
  - – The needle is placed at the base of the prostate, within the junction of the seminal vesicle and the prostate.
  - – The xylocaine is then infiltrated over the entire length of the prostate gland by manually displacing the probe distally within the rectum.
  - – No trials have evaluated a dose–response to different quantities or compositions of anesthesia.

- Inhalational nitrous oxide has been confirmed to ↓ the pain associated with prostate biopsy.
  - – This method may be an option in those patients who cannot tolerate a standard prostate biopsy.
  - – This method is only necessary in rare patients who cannot tolerate placement of the rectal probe.

Number of biopsy cores

- There is no consensus on the optimum number of biopsy cores that should be taken during a routine prostate biopsy.
  - – The false-negative rate of a standard sextant biopsy scheme was ~ 33%.
    [Rabbani F, *J Urol* **159**: 1247–1250,1998]

- Several studies have confirmed the utility of a 12-core biopsy strategy, which ↑ the detection rate of prostate cancer by 20–33%.
  [Levine MA, *J Urol* **159**: 471–476, 1998]
  [Naughton CK, *J Urol* **164**(2): 388–392, 2000]

- Ongoing studies are evaluating the safety and efficacy of additional extended biopsy techniques.

- One technique utilizes up to 24-core biopsies and is termed the 'saturation biopsy technique'.
  [Jones JS, *J Urol* **168**(5): 2108 2110, 2002]
  - There is an ↑ risk of bleeding and infectious complications with this technique.
  - At present there are no data on the incidence of clinically insignificant cancers detected in this group of patients.

Prostate pathology

[Rosai J, *Ackerman's Surgical Pathology*, 8th edn. Mosby-Year Book, Chicago, 1996]
[Sternberg S, *Diagnostic Surgical Pathology*, 3rd edn. Lippincott Williams & Wilkins, Baltimore, OH, 1999]

Prostatic intraepithelial neoplasia

- Low-grade prostatic intraepithelial neoplasia (PIN).
    - Common in young men.
    - Greater architectural complexity than hyperplasia.
    - Occasional enlarged nuclei.
    - Rare nucleoli.
    - Usually diploid.
    - Not reported.
      [Epstein JI, *Am J Surg Pathol* **19**: 873–886, 1995]

- High-grade PIN (HGPIN).
    - Portends increased risk of cancer in subsequent biopsies.
    - Low cancer risk if there are two negative subsequent biopsies.
    - Number of cores with HGPIN predicts risk of subsequent cancer.
    - Present in 80% of carcinomas.
    - Cribriform or micropapillary patterns predict a higher risk of cancer.
      [Kronz JD, *Am J Surg Pathol* **25**: 1079–1085, 2001]
    - Seen in men < 60 years old.
    - More common in black ♂.

- Not associated with increased prostate-specific antigen (PSA).
- If found on transurethral resection of the prostate (TURP), examine all submitted tissue.
- Aneuploid (50%).
- Micropapillary/cribriform (70%).
- Flat/tufted (20%).
- Apocrine/foamy/inverted/mucinous/paneth-cell-like/signet ring/endocrine (10%).
- Frequently multicentric.
- Glands show:
  - Intraluminal papillary projections.
  - May contain cellular pigment/intraluminal mucin.
  - Nucleomegaly.
  - Pleomorphism.
  - Stratification/crowding.
  - Prominent nucleoli.
  - Hyperchromasia.
- Differential diagnosis:
  1. Seminal vesicle glands with cribriform epithelium without atypia.
  2. clear-cell cribriform hyperplasia.
  3. Central zone glands.
    [Srodon M, *Human Pathol* **33**: 518–523, 2002]

- HGPIN with adjacent small atypical glands.
  - Difficult to determine HGPIN vs cancer next to HGPIN.
  - No reliable differentiating features.
  - Higher risk of cancer on repeat biopsy than for HGPIN alone.
  - Patients should be re-biopsied.
    [Kronz JD, *Human Pathol* **32**: 389–395, 2001]

Prostatic carcinoma

Epidemiology

- Most common cancer after skin cancer.
- Second most common cause of death after lung cancer.
- More common and aggressive in black ♂.
- Rare in Asian ♂.

Clinical detection

- Rectal examination, transurethral ultrasound, elevated PSA.

- Firm prostate differential diagnosis:
  1. Granulomatous prostatitis.
  2. Nodular hyperplasia.
  3. Tuberculosis.
  4. Infarct.
  5. Lithiasis.

- Elevated PSA differential diagnosis:
  1. Nodular hyperplasia.
  2. Prostatitis.
  3. Infarct.
  4. Trauma.
  5. Other tumors.
     - Benign disease: increased PSA is usually transient.

Core biopsies

[Varma M, *Arch Pathol Lab Med* **126**: 554–561, 2002]
[Bostwick DG, *Arch Pathol Lab Med* **119**: 444–447, 1995]
[Pacelli A, *Human Pathol* **29**: 543–546, 1998]

- From selected portions of the prostate.

- False-negative results (12%), due to sampling error.

- 25% of specimens with tumor have only a small focus of carcinoma.

- Transrectal biopsies more accurate than transperineal biopsies.

- The Gleason score in biopsy correlates with that in prostatectomy.

- More errors with Gleason scores of 5/6 (underestimates prostatectomy Gleason score).
  [Steinberg DM, *Am J Surg Pathol* **21**: 566–576, 1997]

- Seeding of needle tract is a rare complication of perineal needle biopsy: likely in poorly differentiated carcinoma, less likely in transrectal biopsy.

- Should be reviewed before radical prostatectomy.

- Microscopy:
  - Prominent nucleoli.
  - Marginated nucleoli.
  - Multiple nucleoli.
  - Blue mucin.
  - Intraluminal crystalloids.
  - Perineural invasion.

- Fat invasion.
- Glomerulations.
- Retraction clefts.
- Collagenous micronodules.
- Intraluminal amorphous eosinophilic material.

Minimal prostatic adenocarcinoma on core biopsy

- < 1 mm on biopsy.

- Pathologically significant tumor at prostatectomy.

- Unlikely: perineural invasion, collagenous micronodules, mitotic figures.
  [Thorson P, Mod Pathol 11: 543–551, 1998]

- Differential diagnosis:
  1. Adenosis.
  2. Atrophy.
  3. HGPIN.
     [Thorson P, Am J Clin Pathol 114: 896 909, 2000]

Adenocarcinoma of peripheral ducts and acini

- Distribution.
  [Vargas SO, Am J Clin Pathol 112: 373–376, 1999]
  - 70% in peripheral zone (posterior, lateral, anterior).
  - Early: spares periurethral zone.
  - Posteriorly (> 90%) and anteriorly (65%).
  - Anterior tumors have higher tumor volume and extraprostatic extension.

- Tumor extension.
  - Locally via seminal vesicles and bladder base.
  - Rarely into prostatic urethra or rectum.
  - Potentially as anterior rectal mass, stricture, or serosal implant.

- Metastases.
  - Bones (90%), lung/pleura (46%), liver (25%), adrenal glands (13%).
  - Also lymph nodes, testes, and breast.

- Bone metastasis.
  - Lumbar spine/sacrum/pelvis via Batson's venous plexus.
  - Sequential lumbar to cervical spread.
  - Occurs with small tumors.

- – Multiple, usually osteoblastic.
- – Mimics Paget's disease or osteosarcoma.
- – Causes low calcium/phosphate, and increased alkaline phosphatase.
- – Prostatic alkaline phosphatase (PAP)/PSA (+), even after decalcification.

- Lung metastases.
  - – Small acinar or cribriform growth.
  - – Frequent lymphangitic permeation.
  - – No stromal response.
  - – Uniform round nuclei with prominent nucleoli.
  - – Intraluminal blue mucin (+).
  - – Prominent cell borders.
  - – Usually PSA/PAP (+).
  - – Possible carcinoid-like architecture.
    [Copeland JN, *Am J Clin Pathol* **117**: 552–557, 2002]
  - – Mimics bronchogenic carcinoma.
    [Lee DW, *Am J Clin Pathol* **94**: 641–645, 1990]

- Nodal metastases.
  - – Pelvic chains, then retroperitoneum.
  - – Rarely skips pelvis and goes to lungs/liver.
  - – Mediastinal/left supraclavicular nodes (poorly differentiated).
  - – Rarely in latent cancers diagnosed at autopsy.

- Recurrence after radical prostatectomy.
  - – Median interval 40 months.
  - – Mean tumor size 3.2 mm.
  - – May lack malignant histology.
  - – Atypical glands should not be seen after radical prostatectomy.
    [Ripple MG, *Mod Pathol* **13**: 521–527, 2000]

- Prognostic factors.
  - – Stage.
  - – Gleason score.
  - – Surgical margins.
  - – Preoperative PSA.
    [Bostwick DG, *Arch Pathol Lab Med* **124**: 995–1000, 2000]
  - – Perineurial invasion.
    [Sebo TJ, *Am J Surg Pathol* **26**: 431–439, 2002]
  - – Lymphovascular invasion.
    [Herman CM, *Am J Surg Pathol* **24**: 859–863, 2000]
  - – Nodal metastasis size.
    [Cheng L, *Am J Surg Pathol* **22**: 1491–500, 1998]

- Urinary cytology.
  - Difficult to identify well-differentiated tumors.
  - Easier for poor/moderately differentiated tumors.
  - Not useful for screening (10% false-negative results).
  - Replaced by 18-gauge needle core biopsy.
  - Seminal vesicle cells may resemble cancer.

- Tumor in TURP specimen.
  - Extensive spread by conventional cancer or central cancer.
  - Related to sampling:
    - 5 blocks/12 g (90% detection).
    - 8 blocks/12 g (98% detection).
  - If < 5% carcinoma, sample more chips.
  - If HGPIN only, embed all tissue and obtain deeper level samples.

- Frozen section diagnosis.
  - Look for architectural disarray or perineural invasion.

- Lymph node frozen section/imprints.
  - 10% false-negative results.

- Treatment options.
  - Radical prostatectomy (not warranted if positive pelvic nodes).
  - Brachytherapy (radioactive seeds).
  - External beam radiation therapy.
  - Watchful waiting (low-grade tumors/limited life expectancy).
  - Chemotherapy.
  - Hormone treatment for metastases:
    - Luteinizing hormone releasing hormone (LHRH) analogs.
    - Antiandrogens.
    - Orchiectomy.
  - Tumors are initially androgen sensitive.
  - Monitor response with PSA level.
  - In patients < 20 years old:
    - Carcinoma is rare.
    - Usually obstructive symptoms.
    - Advanced stage.
    - High grade.
    - Poor response to treatment.
    - < 1 year survival.

- Gross.
  - Gritty and firm.
  - Gray-yellow.
  - Poorly delimited.

- More easily felt than seen.
- Often undetectable if tumor small.

- Microscopy.
  - Small glands.
  - Medium-sized glands.
  - Cribriform glands or diffuse, single-cell infiltration with necrosis.
  - Nucleomegaly.
  - Hyperchromasia.
  - Prominent nucleoli (> 3 μm, specific cancer; > 1 μm, suggestive).
  - Mitotic figures extremely rare, except in high-grade tumors.
  - Malignant transformation is accompanied by loss of basal cells.
  - Glands are 'too many, too small, too crowded'.
  - Diagnose carcinoma only if stringent criteria are met.
  - If criteria are not met, then 'atypical glands suspicious for malignancy'.
  - Pattern depends on Gleason grade.

- Common patterns.
  - Infiltrative, medium sized, closely packed glands (Gleason 3) with irregular outline, smooth inner surface, and scanty stroma.
  - Cribriform pattern (Gleason 3, smooth borders; Gleason 4, uneven borders).
  - Single-cell infiltration (Gleason 5, may resemble breast lobular carcinoma).

- Less common patterns.
  - Small, regular, round glands forming expansive nodule (Gleason 1 or 2).
  - Usually not multifocal.
  - Usually in transition or central zone.

- Lymphovascular invasion.
  - Not commonly seen

- Calcifications.
  [Woods JE, *Arch Pathol Lab Med* **122**: 152–155, 1998]
  - More common in benign prostate.
  - May be seen in:
    - Gleason 5, comedo-type necrosis.
    - Gleason 3, intraluminal.
    - Collagenous micronodules.

- Vessel cellularity.
  [Garcia FU, *Mod Pathol* **13**: 717–722, 2000]

- Radical resections with increased vascular cellularity are associated with higher grades.

- Corpora amylacea.
  [Cohen RJ, *Human Pathol* **31**: 94–100, 2000]
  - Benign, but may be found in carcinoma.
  - May arise from release of prostate secretory granules.
  - Do not confuse with crystalloids.

- Crystalloids.
  - Intraluminal eosinophilic rhomboid structures (contain sulfur).
    [Cohen RJ, *Human Pathol* **31**: 94–100, 2000]
  - Present in up to 20% of carcinomas, usually Gleason 3.
  - Rarely in benign glands or metastasis.
    [Molberg KH, *Am J Clin Pathol* **101**: 266–268, 1994]
  - No subsequent significant risk of cancer if found in benign glands.
    [Anton RC, *Am J Surg Pathol* **22**: 446–449, 1998]

- Cytoplasm.
  - Finely granular.
  - May be clear/foamy (intracellular lipid).

- Mucin.
  - Intraluminal acidic mucin (66% of carcinomas).
  - Basophilic or deeply eosinophilic.
  - Normal prostate secretes neutral mucins.
  - Acid mucins also seen in adenosis and after radiation therapy.

- Perineural invasion.
  - In up to 85% of carcinomas.
  - If present, suggests extraprostatic extension.
    [Vargas SO, *Am J Clin Pathol* **111**: 223–228, 1999]
  - Diameter of invasion may be a prognostic factor.
    [Maru N, *Human Pathol* **32**: 828–833, 2001]
  - Cancer expresses nerve cell adhesion factor that may propagate spread.
    [Li R, *Human Pathol* **34**: 457–461, 2003]
  - Outdated theories:
    - Spread via perineural lymphatic system.
    - Perineurial space is the tissue plane of least resistance.

- Features diagnostic of adenocarcinoma.
  - Perineural invasion.
  - Glomerulation.
  - Mucinous fibroplasia.
    [Baisden BL, *Am J Surg Pathol* **23**: 918–924, 1999]

- Features favoring diagnosis of adenocarcinoma.
  - Small glands between larger glands.
  - Crowded glands.
  - Prominent nucleoli.
  - Nuclear enlargement.
  - Hyperchromatic nuclei.
  - Amphophilic cytoplasm.
  - Mitotic figures.
  - Blue luminal mucin.
  - Pink luminal mucin.
  - Crystalloids.
  - Adjacent HGPIN.

- Warning features.
  - Atrophic cytoplasm.
  - Atypical glands associated with inflammation.
  - Small, crowded glands merging with large, benign glands (adenosis).
  - Small, crowded glands with corpora amylacea (adenosis).
  - Small, atypical, crowded glands adjacent to HGPIN (tangential HGPIN).

- Grading (Gleason).
  [Rubin MA, Am J Surg Pathol **24**: 1634–1640, 2000]
  - Grades 1–5, based on glandular differentiation.
  - Score 2–10, based on grade for first and second most common patterns.
  - If only one pattern seen, first and second patterns are given the same grade.
  - Score 2–4 (well differentiated) almost never develop aggressive disease.
  - Score 8–10 usually die of disease.
  - Clinically important distinctions are Gleason scores 2–6, 7, 8, and 9–10.
  - Upgrading is seen in 1/3 of prostatectomy specimens after biopsy.
  - Down-grading is seen in 5% of prostatectomy specimens after biopsy.
  - 1/3 of Gleason 8 at biopsy are Gleason 7 at radical prostatectomy.
  - If there is minimal tumor on biopsy (< 1 mm), the Gleason score does not predict tumor stage.

- Gleason grades.
  - Grade 1.
    - Single, separate, closely packed, uniform, round glands arranged in a circumscribed nodule with pushing borders.

- – Uncommon pattern, except in transitional zone adenocarcinomas.
- – Almost never seen in needle biopsies.

- Grade 2.
  - – More variability in gland shape, and more stroma separating glands.
  - – Less circumscribed at periphery.
  - – Not infiltrative.
  - – Common in transitional zone tumors.
  - – Infrequent in peripheral zone tumors.
  - – Usually periurethral and not sampled.

- Gleason grades 1 or 2 are not diagnosed on core biopsies since:
  - – They are uncommon in the peripheral zone.
  - – There is marked interpathologist variability.
  - – Usually reflects undergrading compared with experts.
  - – Does not correlate with radical prostatectomy.

- Grade 3.
  - – Single, separate, much more variable glands.
  - – May be closely packed, but usually are irregularly separated.
  - – Slightly infiltrative.
  - – Tangentially cut glands may be poorly formed.
  - – Patterns:
    - – Well-formed, angulate/compressed glands infiltrating benign glands.
    - – Small but separate glands with inconspicuous lumen.
    - – Papillary or cribriform; difficult to differentiate from cribriform PIN.
      [Kronz JD, *Am J Surg Pathol* **25**: 147–155, 2001]
    - – Large-gland variant.

- Grade 4.
  - – Fused glands lacking stroma and fragmenting easily.
  - – Patterns:
    - – Small acinar glands fusing into cords/chains.
    - – Some well-formed lumina.
    - – Papillary–cribriform.
    - – Hypernephroid pattern.

- Grade 5.
  - – Predicts early death.
    [Vollmer RT, *Am J Clin Pathol* **116**: 864–870, 2001]

- Patterns:
  - 5a: comedocarcinoma–papillary/cribriform, with central necrosis.
  - 5b: minimal gland formation, infiltrating single cells/solid sheet.

- Atypical glands, suspicious for malignancy.
  - Diagnosed in 5% of biopsies.
  - Do not fulfill complete criteria for malignancy due to:
    - Small size of the focus.
    - Small number of cells with enlarged nucleoli.
    - Clustered growth pattern.
    - Presence of HGPIN within many foci.
  - With more sampling up to 60% show carcinoma.
    [Cheville JC, *Am J Clin Pathol* **108**: 633–640, 1997]
  - Back off diagnosis if associated with a few neutrophils.
  - Most tumors outside the central zone are multifocal in radical prostatectomies.
  - Fibroblastic nuclei surrounding obvious cancer may mimic basal cells.

- Minimal residual cancer at radical prostatectomy.
  [DiGiuseppe JA, *Am J Surg Pathol* **21**: 174–178, 1997]
  - 3–4% of cases.
  - Review of initial biopsies in cases with no residual cancer showed:
    - Cancer confirmation.
    - HGPIN only.
    - Mislabeled specimen.

Immunohistochemistry

- High molecular weight cytokeratin (HMWK).
  - Basal-cell-specific, anti-keratin antibody.
  - Adenocarcinomas do not stain.
  - Internal positive control of benign glands must be seen.
  - Negative HMWK is diagnostic of cancer only if there is high morphologic pre-test suspicion.
  - Positive staining identifies mimickers of cancer:
    - Benign crowded glands.
    - Adenosis.
    - Atrophy.
    - Differentiate HGPIN vs cancer.

- False negative results (5%) in:
  - Inflamed acini.
  - Atypical adenomatous hyperplasia.
  - Post-atrophic hyperplasia.
  - Atrophy.
  - HGPIN.
  - Basal cell carcinoma.
  - Adenoid cystic carcinoma (fragmented or continuous staining).

- Prostate specific antigen (PSA)/prostatic alkaline phosphatase (PAP).
  [Feiner HD, *Am J Surg Pathol* **11**: 765–770, 1986]
  [Mai KT, *Human Pathol* **27**: 1377–1381, 1996]
  - Positive in tumor and benign cells.
  - Identifies prostatic origin of most metastatic tumors.
  - Differentiates between prostatic and urothelial carcinomas.
  - PSA more sensitive and specific than PAP.
  - PSA/PAP less sensitive in poorly differentiated adenocarcinoma.
  - May become (–) after hormone treatment.
  - Non-prostate tumors usually are negative or weak with PSA/PAP.

- α-Methylacyl-coenzyme A racemase (AMACR (P504S))
  [Beach R, *Am J Surg Pathol* **26**: 1588–1596, 2002]
  [Jiang Z, *Am J Surg Pathol* **25**: 1397–1404, 2001]
  - Protein involved in branched chain, fatty acid metabolism.
  - Sensitive and specific for prostate cancer.
  - Positive in some hyperplastic nodules and benign glands next to transition zone carcinomas.
  - Use AMACR/HMWK combination to diagnose limited prostatic carcinoma.

Other prostate carcinomas

- **Adenoid basal cell tumor**.
  - Resembles the salivary gland tumor.
  - Usually does not develop progressive disease; expansive growth pattern.
  - Clustered, multinodular, basaloid cells, some with punched out lumens.
  - Fibromyxoid stroma.
  - Squamous differentiation.
  - Basal cell hyperplasia background.
  - HMWK (+), p63 (+), PSA (–), PAP (–).
    [Young RH, *Am J Clin Pathol* **89**: 49–56, 1988]

- **Adenosquamous carcinoma.**
  - De novo, post-radiation or hormone therapy for ordinary adeno-carcinoma.
  [Moyana TN, *Am J Surg Pathol* **11**: 403–407, 1987]

- **Atrophic adenocarcinoma.**
  - Malignant acini that architecturally resemble atrophy/post-atrophic hyperplasia.
  - Retains cytologic cancerous features.
  - Not associated with hormone therapy.
  - Round dilated/distorted acini lined by attenuated epithelium with scant cytoplasm.
  - Infiltrative growth pattern.
  - Nucleomegaly and prominent nucleoli.
  - Atrophic features in 25% of total tumor in biopsies and prosta-tectomies.
  - Usually Gleason score 6–7.
  [Cina SJ, *Am J Surg Pathol* **21**: 289–295, 1997]

- **Basaloid carcinoma.**
  [Yang XJ, *Human Pathol* **29**: 1447–1450, 1998]
  - Very rare; either variably highly aggressive or low malignant potential.
  - Desmoplastic stromal response.
  - Perineural, widespread infiltration, and necrosis.
  - bcl-2 (+), Ki-67 (+).
  [Yang XJ, *Human Pathol* **29**: 1447–50, 1998]
  - Differential diagnosis: basal cell hyperplasia, bcl-2 (–) and Ki-67 (–).

- **Carcinosarcoma.**
  [Lauwers GY, *Am J Surg Pathol* **17**: 342–349, 1993]
  - Rare.
  - Adenocarcinoma with sarcomatoid transformation.
  - Biphasic tumor with adenocarcinoma and sarcoma elements.
  - Can be related to radiotherapy or hormone therapy.
  - Sarcoma component: PSA (–), EMA (–), keratin (–).

- **Clear-cell adenocarcinoma.**
  [Pan CC, *Am J Surg Pathol* **24**: 1433–1436, 2000]
  - Extremely rare.
  - More common in urethra/bladder.
  - Well-circumscribed lesion with tubulocystic/papillary glands.
  - Glycogen-rich, cuboidal/hobnail cells with clear/eosinophilic cytoplasm.
  - Resembles ovarian neoplasm.

- Keratin (+), EMA (+), focal HMWK (+), PSA (–), PAP(–).
- Differential diagnosis: urothelial and renal cell carcinoma.

- **Foamy gland adenocarcinoma.**
  [Tran TT, *Am J Surg Pathol* **25**: 618–623, 2001]
  - Rare variant with abundant foamy cytoplasm and minimal cytologic atypia.
  - Large bilateral tumor with extraprostatic extension.
  - Has intracytoplasmic vesicles (no lipid or neutral mucin).
  - Aggressive behavior.
  - AMACR (+), mucicarmine (–).
  - Differential diagnosis:
    1. Mucinous metaplasia: mucicarmine (+).
    2. Cowper's glands: ducts embedded in skeletal muscle.
    3. Clear-cell cribriform hyperplasia.
    4. Gleason hypernephroid pattern 4.

- **Lymphoepithelial-like carcinoma.**
  - Resembles nasopharyngeal lymphoepithelial-like carcinoma.
  - HLA-DR (+).

- **Mucinous (colloid) adenocarcinoma.**
  - Uncommon (< 1%).
  - Intra- and extracellular mucin must comprise 25% of tumor.
  - May be more hormone independent.
  - Less responsive to radiation therapy.
  - Aggressive biologic behavior.
    [Epstein JI, *Am J Surg Pathol* **9**: 299–308, 1985]
  - Tumor cells float in pools of mucin; rare signet ring cells.
  - PSA (+), PAP (+).
  - Patterns:
    - Microglandular.
    - Cribriform.
    - Hypernephroid.
    - Solid.
    - Comedo.
  - Differential diagnosis:
    1. Colonic cancer extension.
    2. Bladder mucinous adenocarcinoma: PSA (–), PAP (–).
    3. Cowper's gland carcinoma.

- **Mucinous adenocarcinoma from prostatic urethra–urinary bladder type.**
  [Tran KP, *Am J Surg Pathol* **20**: 1346–1350, 1996]

- Very rare.
- Confined to prostate and originating from prostatic urethra.
- Identical to adenocarcinomas arising within the urinary bladder.
- Different from mucinous adenocarcinoma of the prostate.
- In situ adenocarcinoma component present in overlying prostatic urethra.
- Mucin lakes with tall columnar epithelium and variable cytologic atypia.
- CEA (+), PSA (–), PAP (–).

- **Neuroendocrine carcinoma.**
  [Wynn SS, *Arch Pathol Lab Med* **124**: 1074–1076, 2000]
  - Neuroendocrine cells found in 80% of normal prostates.
  - Poorer prognosis.
  - More resistant to hormone therapy.
  - Pure neuroendocrine carcinomas not associated with elevated PSA.
  - May resemble Paneth cells and typical/atypical carcinoid.
  - Chromogranin (+), PSA (+), PAP (+), bcl-2 (±), ACTH (±), β-endorphin (±), calcitonin (±).

- **Pseudohyperplastic adenocarcinoma**.
  [Levi AW, *Am J Surg Pathol* **24**: 1039–1046, 2000]
  - Rare, resembles benign hyperplastic glands.
  - Not a low-grade lesion as is associated with Gleason scores 5–7.
  - Difficult to grade; defer grade for radical prostatectomy.
  - Papillary infoldings, crowded glands, large atypical glands, nucleomegaly, pink amorphous secretions, occasional to frequent nucleoli, branching, and crystalloids.
  - HMFK (–), AMACR (+).
    [Zhou M, *Am J Surg Pathol* **27**: 772–778, 2003]
  - Differential diagnosis: adenosis and HGPIN.

- **Prostatic duct carcinoma.**
  - < 1% of prostatic carcinomas.
  - Usually periurethral, but can be seen in the peripheral zone.
  - Often near the verumontanum.
  - Associated with obstructive symptoms and hematuria.
  - Usually diagnosed on TURP.
  - May have normal digital rectal examination and normal PSA.
  - Usually aggressive and less likely to respond to hormone therapy.
  - Presents at higher stage.
    [Brinker DA, *Am J Surg Pathol* **23**: 1471–1479, 1999]
  - 80% have a small acinar component and thus may represent peripheral zone adenocarcinomas infiltrating into large periurethral

ducts and stroma, and not represent a distinct histologic type.
[Bock BJ, *Am J Surg Pathol* **23**: 781–785, 1999]

- Papillary or cribriform pattern with slit-like lumina or discrete glands lined with tall, pseudostratified epithelium with abundant, amphophilic cytoplasm.
- May have pale/clear cytoplasm; stromal fibrosis.
- May have pagetoid spread throughout the prostatic urethra or intraluminally within ducts before invading the surrounding stroma.
  [Samaratunga H, *Am J Surg Pathol* **21**: 435–440, 1997]
- The presence of basal cells does not exclude these tumors.
- HMWK (+) in cribriforming ductal adenocarcinoma and other patterns, PSA (+), PAP (+).
- Differential diagnosis: HGPIN vs cribriform pattern of duct carcinoma.

- **Signet ring carcinoma.**
  [Alguacil-Garcia A, *Am J Surg Pathol* **10**: 795–800, 1986]
  [Alline KM, *Arch Pathol Lab Med* **116**: 99–102, 1992]
  [Ro JY, *Am J Surg Pathol* **12**: 453–460, 1988]
  [Torbenson M, *Mod Pathol* **11**: 552–559, 1998]
  [Wang HL, *Am J Surg Pathol* **26**: 1066–1070, 2002]
  - Rare, highly malignant.
  - Solid, acinar, single-line patterns.
  - Tumor cells with signet ring pattern (at least 25%) due to intracellular mucin.
  - PSA (+) (variable in some studies), AE1/AE3 (+), CAM 5.2 (+), mucicarmine (±).
  - Differential diagnosis:
    1. Artifact in lymphocytes.
    2. Benign signet ring change.

- **Small-cell carcinoma.**
  - Pure or combined with ductal carcinoma.
  - May cause Cushing's syndrome and/or syndrome of inappropriate antidiuretic hormone (SIADH).
  - Some have endocrine features.
  - Very aggressive; cannot monitor with PSA.
  - Survival usually < 1 year.
    [Bleichner JC, *Arch Pathol Lab Med* **110**: 1041–1044, 1986]
  - Associated with limbic encephalitis.
    [Stern RC, *Mod Pathol* **12**: 814–818, 1999]
  - Resembles lung small-cell carcinoma with apoptotic bodies.
  - Chromogranin (+), NSE (+), TTF-1 (±).
    [Agoff SN, *Mod Pathol* **13**: 238–242, 2000]
  - PSA (−), PAP (−).

- **Squamous cell carcinoma.**
  - Extremely rare.
  - De novo or after estrogen therapy, flutamine therapy, or brachy-therapy.
  - Poor survival.
  - Osteolytic metastases.
  - Does not respond to hormone therapy.
  - No ↑ PSA with metastases.

- **Urothelial carcinoma (primary).**
  [Bassily NH, *Am J Surg Pathol* **113**: 383–388, 2000]
  - < 2% of primary tumors.
  - Arises from periurethral duct urothelium.
  - Looks identical to bladder tumors.
  - Invades bladder neck and soft tissue.
  - 20% have distant metastases to bone (osteolytic), lung, and liver.
  - Poor prognosis, even when in situ only.
  - Treatment: cystoprostatectomy, chemotherapy, and radiation.
  - In cystoprostatectomies for urothelial cancer, 50% have prostate cancer.
  - In situ carcinoma usually present.
  - Nests of neoplastic cells filling prostatic ducts with comedo necrosis.
  - Stromal invasion with small cell nests, with anaplasia and many with mitosis.
  - PSA (–), PAP (–), CK7 (+), CK20 (±), CEA (±).
    [Genega EM, *Mod Pathol* **13**: 1186–1191, 2000]
    [Mhawech P, *Human Pathol* **33**: 1136–1140, 2002]
  - Differential diagnosis:
    - Bladder extension of urethral carcinoma.
    - High-grade urothelial vs high-grade prostate carcinoma.

Sarcoma, lymphoma, and other malignancies

- **Angiosarcoma.**
  [Chandan VS, *Arch Pathol Lab Med* **127**: 876–878, 2003]
  - Rare in the prostate.
  - Potentially radiation induced years after carcinoma treatment.
  - Proliferative vessels lined by atypical, multilayered to solid endo-thelial cells.
  - Tumor cells pleomorphic, variably spindled to large/plump.
  - Pleomorphic nuclei with clumped chromatin and prominent nucleoli.

- Frequent mitotic figures, some atypical.
- CD31 (+), CD34 (+), factor VIII (+), PSA (–), keratin (–).

- **Leiomyosarcoma.**
  - Causes obstruction, involves adjacent organs.
  - Most common sarcoma in adults.
  - Mean survival 3–4 years
  - Tends to recur.
  - Metastases to liver and lung.
  - Desmin (+), h-caldesmon (+).
  - Differential diagnosis:
    1. Nodular hyperplasia with atypical changes.
    2. Postoperative spindle cell nodules.

- **Embryonal rhabdomyosarcoma.**
  - Most common malignant tumor in children/infants.
  - Firm, smooth enlargement of the prostate.
  - Nodal metastasis is less common than when this tumor is in the head and neck.
  - Usually presents with stage 3 disease.
  - Sometimes there are distant metastases.
  - 80% of patients are cured; most stage 4 patients die of disease.
  - Prognosis: better if there is a leiomyosarcoma-like appearance.
  - Treatment: multiple-agent chemotherapy, surgery, and radiation.
  - Micro: cellular, particularly around blood vessels, alternating with myxoid/edematous areas and necrosis; small round/oval/spindly tumor cells; may have bizarre forms with abundant, eosinophilic cytoplasm, variable cross-striations; usually extraprostatic extension.
  - Desmin (+), myogenin (+).
  - Differential diagnosis: bladder rhabdomyosarcoma.

- **Lymphoma.**
  - 10% of non-Hodgkin's lymphoma and 10% of leukemias (20% of chronic lymphatic leukemia (CLL)) involve the prostate.
  - 1% of pelvic nodes are removed at prostatectomy (CLL usually).
  - Rarely, is the initial site for Hodgkin's or angiotropic lymphoma.
  - Small lymphocytic leukemia (SLL) may be incidentally identified in pelvic lymph nodes.
    [Weir EG, *Arch Pathol Lab Med* **127**: 567–572, 2003]
  - Micro-SLL: diffuse architectural effacement, tumor effaces sinuses, pseudo-follicles present, no cortical follicles.

- **Perivascular epithelioid cell tumor (PEComa).**
  - Include:
    - Clear-cell, 'sugar' tumor of the lung.

- Lymphangiomyomatosis.
- Angiomyolipoma.
- Epithelioid cells with clear/granular cytoplasm in perivascular fashion.
- HMB45 (+), MelanA/MART1 (variable +), keratin (–), S100 (–).
- Differential diagnosis: clear-cell sarcoma of soft parts (S100 (+)).
[Pan CC, *Arch Pathol Lab Med* **127**: E96–E98, 2003]

- **Primitive peripheral neuroectodermal tumor (PNET).**
  - Rare and aggressive.
  [Colecchia M, *Arch Pathol Lab Med* **127**: e190–e193, 2003]
  - Solid nests/sheets of small, round cells.
  - CD99/MIC2 (+), vimentin (+), NSE (+), synaptophysin (+).
  - EWS/FLI1 type 2 chimeric transcript.
  - Differential diagnosis:
    1. Small-cell carcinoma: CD99 (–).
    2. Rhabdomyosarcoma: desmin (+).
    3. Lymphoma (lymphoblastic lymphoma): CD99 (+), TdT (+).
    4. Desmoplastic, small, round-cell tumor: keratin (+), desmin (+), WT1 (+).

- **Solitary fibrous tumor.**
  - Rare and often misdiagnosed.
  - Some cases have malignant behavior.
  - Collagenization, hemangiopericytoma-like, spindled cells between strips of collagen.
  - CD34 (+), keratin (–).
  [Pins MR, *Arch Pathol Lab Med* **125**: 274–277, 2001]

- **Stromal proliferation of uncertain malignant potential.**
  - May resemble breast phyllodes tumors.
  - May recur rapidly after resection and progress to stromal sarcoma.
  - Patterns:
    - Hypercellular stroma with scattered cytologically atypical cells, associated with benign glands.
    - Hypercellular stroma with minimal cytological atypia, associated with benign glands.
    - Hypercellular stroma with or without cytologically atypical cells, associated with benign glands in a 'leaf-like' growth pattern that resembles phyllodes tumors of the mammary gland.
    - Hypercellular stroma without cytologically atypical stromal cells and without glands.
    [Gaudin PB, *Am J Surg Pathol* **22**: 148–162, 1998]

- Differential diagnosis:
  1. Stromal sarcomas.
  2. Phyllodes tumors.

- **Stromal sarcomas.**
  - Mean age of presentation 54 years.
  - Present with urinary retention, hematuria, hematospermia, rectal mass.
  - Includes phyllodes tumors.
  - Greater cellularity, mitoses, necrosis, and stromal overgrowth than in tumors of 'uncertain malignant potential'.
  - Either pure stromal elements or stromal elements with benign glands resembling malignant breast phyllodes tumors.
  - Positive markers: vimentin (100%), CD34 (100%), PR (85%), desmin (50%), smooth-muscle actin (33%), HHF-35 (25%).
  - Negative stains: S100 (100%), ER (usually).
  - Differential diagnosis: stromal proliferation of uncertain malignant potential.

- **Synovial sarcoma.**
  - Uniform spindle and oval cells forming interlacing fascicles.
  - Hypocellular myxoid.
  - Pericytomatous.
  - EMA (focal (+)), keratin (focal (+)).
  - Negative stains: S100, keratin, NSE, CD34, desmin, MSA, SMA.
  - Molecular: t(X;18).
  [Iwasaki H, *Am J Surg Pathol* 23: 220–226, 1999]

- **Seminal vesicles carcinoma.**
  [Tanaka T, *Human Pathol* 18: 200–202,1987]
  [Ormsby AH, *Mod Pathol* 13: 46–51, 2000]
  - Very rare.
  - Should be localized primarily to seminal vesicle.
  - Must rule out invasion from prostate, rectum, or other site.
  - Should preferable be a papillary adenocarcinoma.
  - Resembles Gleason patterns 3 or 4, prostatic duct adenocarcinoma, or mucinous carcinoma.
  - Usually unresectable and patients die within 2 years.
  - CK7 (+), CA-125 (+), PSA (–), PAP (–), CK20 (–).
  - Differential diagnosis:
    - Prostatic adenocarcinoma: PSA (+), PAP (+), CA-125 (–).
    - Bladder urothelial carcinoma: CK20 (+), CA-125 (–), CK7 (+).
    - Rectal adenocarcinoma: CA-125 (–), CK7 (–), CK20 (+).
    - Bladder adenocarcinoma: CA-125 (–), CK7 (–), CK20 (+).

- **Tumors extending directly into the prostate.**
  - Bladder.
  - Urethra.
  - Colorectum.
  - Anus.
  - Soft tissue tumors.

- **Tumors metastatic to the prostate.**
  - Uncommon.
  - Lung tumors and melanomas predominate.

CHAPTER 9

Staging

[Greene FL, *AJCC Cancer Staging Manual*, 6th edn. Springer-Verlag, New York, 2002, pp. 309–316]

Clinical

- Digital rectal examination is the most common modality utilized to define the local stage.

- Transrectal ultrasound is also utilized.
  - Limited ability to define location and extent of disease.

- Clinically suspicious areas of the prostate should be confirmed histologically by needle biopsies.

- Less commonly, detection occurs at the time of histological analysis of prostate tissue 'chips' from transurethral resection of the prostate.

Pathologic

- Prostatoseminal–vesiculectomy, including regional lymph node sampling and histologic confirmation, is required for pathologic T staging.
  - Exceptions: positive rectal biopsy (pT_4), positive seminal vesicle biopsy or positive biopsy of extraprostatic soft tissue (pT_3).

TNM classification

Primary tumor (T)

Clinical

T_X Primary tumor cannot be assessed.

T_0 No evidence of primary tumor.

T_1 Clinically inapparent tumor neither palpable nor visible by imaging.

T_{1a} Tumor incidental histologic finding in $\leq$ 5% of resected tissue.

T_{1b} Tumor incidental histologic finding in > 5% of resected tissue.

T_{1c} Tumor identified by needle biopsy (e.g. because of elevated prostate-specific antigen (PSA)).

T_2 Tumor confined within the prostate.*

T_{2a} Tumor involves one-half of one lobe or less.

T_{2b} Tumor involves more than one-half of one lobe, but not both lobes.

T_{2c} Tumor involves both lobes.

T_3 Tumor extends through the prostate capsule.†

T_{3a} Extracapsular extension (unilateral or bilateral).

T_{3b} Tumor invades seminal vesicle(s).

T_4 Tumor is fixed or invades adjacent structures other than seminal vesicles: bladder neck, external sphincter, rectum, levator muscles, and/or pelvic wall.

*Tumor found in one or both lobes by needle biopsy, but not palpable or reliably visible by imaging, is classified as T_{1c}.

†Invasion into the prostatic apex or into (but not beyond) the prostatic capsule is classified not as T_3 but as T_2.

Pathologic (pT)

pT_2 Organ confined.*

pT_{2a} Unilateral, involving one-half of one lobe or less.

pT_{2b} Unilateral, involving more than one-half of one lobe, but not both lobes.

pT_{2c} Bilateral disease.

pT_3 Extraprostatic extension.

pT_{3a} Extraprostatic extension.†

pT_{3b} Seminal vesicle invasion.

pT_4 Invasion of bladder, rectum.

*There is no pathologic T_1 classification due to insufficient tissue to determine the highest pT category.

†Positive surgical margin should be indicated by an R_1 descriptor (residual microscopic disease).

Regional lymph nodes (N)

- Nodes of the true pelvis below the bifurcation of the common iliac arteries: pelvic not otherwise specified (NOS), hypogastric, obturator, iliac (internal, external, or NOS), sacral (lateral presacral, promontory (Gerota's), or NOS).
  - Laterality does not affect the N classification.

- Clinical.
  N_X Regional lymph nodes were not assessed.
  N_0 No regional lymph node metastasis.
  N_1 Metastasis in regional lymph node(s).

- Pathological.
  pN_X Regional nodes not sampled.
  pN_0 No positive regional nodes.
  pN_1 Metastasis in regional node(s).

Distant metastasis (M)*

M_X Distant metastasis cannot be assessed (not evaluated by any modality).
M_0 No distant metastasis.
M_1 Distant metastasis.
M_{1a} Non-regional lymph nodes: aortic (para-aortic lumbar), common iliac, deep inguinal, superficial inguinal (femoral), supraclavicular, cervical, scalene, retroperitoneal NOS.
M_{1b} Bone(s).
M_{1c} Other site(s) with or without bone disease.

*When more than one site of metastasis is present, the most advanced category (pM_{1c}) is used.

Histologic grade (G)

G_X Grade cannot be assessed.
G_1 Well differentiated (slight anaplasia) (Gleason 2–4).
G_2 Moderate differentiated (moderate anaplasia) (Gleason 5–6).
G_{3-4} Poorly differentiated/undifferentiated (marked anaplasia) (Gleason 7–10).

- Gleason score assigns a number from 1 to 5 for the two most prevalent histological patterns in the prostate tissue being evaluated to yield a number from 2 to 10.
  - If only one focus of tumor is seen, the number should be assigned twice (i.e. if one focus of Gleason 2 is seen, the Gleason score is 2 + 2).

Stage grouping

Stage I	T_{1a}	N_0	M_0	G_1
Stage II	T_{1a}	N_0	M_0	$G_{2, 3-4}$
	T_{1b}	N_0	M_0	Any G
	T_{1c}	N_0	M_0	Any G
	T_1	N_0	M_0	Any G
	T_2	N_0	M_0	Any G
Stage III	T_3	N_0	M_0	Any G
Stage IV	T_4	N_0	M_0	Any G
	Any T	N_1	M_0	Any G
	Any T	Any N	M_1	Any G

Radiological evaluation

[Scherr D, National Comprehensive Cancer Network Guidelines for the management of prostate cancer. *Urology* **61** (Suppl 2A): 14–24, 2003]

- Bone scan recommended only for patients with one or more of the following:
  - PSA level > 10 ng/ml.
  - Gleason score ≥ 8.
  - Symptomatic bone pain consistent with metastatic disease.
  - Clinical T_3 or T_4 prostate cancer.
- Previous reports indicate positive bone scan results in < 1% of patients whose PSA level is < 10 ng/ml.
  [Lee CT, *Urol Clin North Am* **24**: 389–394, 1997]

- Computerized tomography (CT) or magnetic resonance imaging (MRI) recommended for:
  [Huncharek M, *Abdom Imaging* **21**: 364–367, 1996]
  - Detection of lymph node involvement in patients with T_3 or T_4 disease.
  - Patients who are predicted to have > 20% likelihood of lymph node involvement according to nomogram predictions.

- Fine-needle aspiration may be used to biopsy clinically suspicious enlarged lymph nodes.
  - Rarely are lymph nodes grossly enlarged when PSA < 20 ng/ml, resulting in a low positive predictive value of CT or MRI.

10

Prognostic factors and predictive factors in prostate cancer

[Bostwick DG, *Arch Pathol Lab Med* **124**: 995–1000, 2000]
[Hamdy FC, *Cancer Treat Rev* **27**: 143–151, 2001]
[Feneley MR, *Curr Opin Urol* **10**(4): 319–327, 2000]

- A **prognostic factor** is capable of providing information on clinical outcome at the time of diagnosis, independent of therapy.

- A **predictive factor** is capable of providing information on the likelihood of response to a given therapeutic modality.
  - To understand predictive factors, subgroup analyses are acquired, but these have to be substantiated and validated.
  - Currently, there are no predictive factors or markers that are utilized in prostate carcinoma.
  - Androgen receptor status in prostate carcinoma does not predict response to hormone therapy.

- **Clinical prognostic factors**:
  - Serum prostate-specific antigen (PSA).
  - Gleason score.
  - Digital rectal examination (DRE).
  - Extent of tumor on systemic prostate biopsy.

- **Pathological markers**:
  [Bostwick DG, *Arch Pathol Lab Med* **124**: 995–1000, 2000]
  [*Prognostic Factors for Prostate Cancer*, College of American Pathologists and World Health Organization]
  - Category I: recommended for routine reporting.
    - TNM stage.

- Histological grade (Gleason).
- Surgical margin status.
- Perioperative serum PSA.
- Category II: factors with promise or recommended despite incomplete data.
    - DNA ploidy.
    - Histologic type.
    - Tumor amount in needle biopsy tissue (recommended).
    - Tumor amount in radical prostatectomy specimens (recommended).
- Category III: not currently recommended due to insufficient evidence.
    - Genetic markers.
    - Neuroendocrine markers.
    - Proliferation markers, apoptosis.
    - Perineural invasion.
    - Vascular/lymphatic invasion.
    - Microvessel density.
    - Nuclear morphometry.
    - Androgen receptors.

Serum prostate-specific antigen

- PSA is a serine protease and organ-specific glycoprotein (molecular weight 34,000 Da) which originates in the cytoplasm of the ductal cells of the prostate.

- PSA is tissue-specific but not tumor-specific in the prostate.

- The measurement of serum PSA concentrations is now well established as a useful investigation in the diagnosis and follow-up of patients with prostate cancer.

- PSA concentrations are the best overall predictor of bone-scan findings and can be used as a screening test for prostate cancer.

- Several studies report various optimum cut-off levels, largely due to the different nature of the assays used.

- Recent evidence suggests that the PSA ratio inversely correlates with the aggressiveness of prostate cancer and has the potential to predict tumor grade.

- Controversy regarding PSA as a screening test.

- Recommendations against PSA screening have been issued by the US Preventive Services Task Force, the Canadian Task Force on the Periodic Health Examination, and the Canadian Urologic Association.
  [Woolf SH, *N Engl J Med* **333**(21): 1401–1405, 1995]

- The overall benefit of monitoring PSA after treatment with surgery or radiation therapy for non-metastatic prostate cancer remains controversial.
  [Vicini FA, *J Urol* **173**: 1456–1462, 2005]

- The toxicity of administering salvage therapies of uncertain efficacy after biochemical failure needs to be evaluated to determine the appropriate use of this marker.

- PSA doubling time (PSADT) pretreatment has been examined as a predictor of post-treatment failure after radiation therapy.
  - Patients with a PSADT < 12 months had a 50% failure rate by 18 months.
  - Patients with a PSADT that did not ↑ demonstrated only a 3% failure at 3 years.
    [Hanks GE, *Int J Radiat Oncol Biol Phys* **34**: 549–553, 1996]

- Various kinetic parameters of PSA, such as the PSADT, time to PSA recurrence, and PSA velocity, have been used to try to predict local vs distant recurrences after radical prostatectomy.
  - A PSADT after radical prostatectomy of < 6 months correlated with distant metastases, and a PASDT of > 6 months correlated with local failure.
    [Patel A, *J Urol* **158**: 1441–1445, 1997]
    [Roberts SG, *Mayo Clin Proc* **76**: 576–581, 2001]

Digital rectal examination

[Partin AW, *J Urol* **150**: 110,1993]

- Experience is very important.

- Sensitivity in predicating organ-confined cancer is approximately 50%; the specificity is 80%.

Gleason score

[Humphrey PA, *Mod Pathol* **17**: 292–306, 2004]

- This technique was developed by Dr Donald F. Gleason and members

of the Veterans Administration Cooperative Urological Research Group (VACURG).
- From 1960 to 1975 the VACURG enrolled ~ 5,000 prostate cancer patients in prospective, randomized, clinical trials.

- One of the outstanding strengths of the Gleason grading system is that it was tested in this large patient population, with long-term follow-up that included use of survival as an endpoint.
  - The assignment of a Gleason score, which is the addition of the two most common patterns, essentially averages the primary and secondary grades.

- The grading system is based entirely on the histologic pattern of the arrangement of carcinoma cells in hematoxylin and eosin (H&E) stained sections.

Surgical margin status

- For patients with organ-confined disease, (+) margins are associated with higher rates of PSA progression.
  [Blute ML, *Cancer* **82**: 902–908, 1998]

- (+) margins and biochemical failure rates are similar or identical for the perineal and retropubic approaches for organ-confined prostate cancer.
  [Boccon-Gibod L, *J Urol* **160**: 1383–1385, 1998]
  - The perineal approach is associated with a significantly ↑ risk of capsular incisions and surgically induced (+) margins, and thus an ↑ risk of biochemical failure.
  - A regression analysis analyzing the effect of Gleason score, distance between tumor and margin, location of closest margin, and pathological stage as related to progression.
    [Epstein JI, *J Urol* **157**: 241–243, 1997]
  - RESULTS:
    - Only grade was predictive of progression ($p < 0.00001$).
    - Patients with progression were no more likely to have tumor close to the margin than were those without progression.

- Between 1987 and 1993, 423 cases could be identified with clinical stage T_{1-2} prostate cancer treated with radical prostatectomy.
  [Kupelian PA, *Int J Radiat Oncol Biol Phys* **37**: 1043–1052, 1997]
  - The 5-year biochemical relapse-free survival rates for margin (+) vs margin (–) patients were 37% and 78%, respectively.

- Recurrence and progression correlated with the number of surgical margins involved by tumor, pathological Gleason score, and baseline pre-prostatectomy PSA levels.
  [Lowe BA, J Urol **158**: 1452–1456, 1997]
  - PSA recurrence was seen in 20.8% (10/48) patients with 1 surgical margin involved, 40.9% (9/22) with 2 margins involved, and 50% (5/10) with ≥ 3 margins involved.

- The interval to progression (↑ PSA level) was measured in 478 ♂ by status of the surgical margins.
  [Ohori M, J Urol **154**: 1818–1824, 1995]
  - RESULTS:
    - At 5 years, the non-progression rate was 64% for patients with and 83% for those without (+) surgical margins.
    - With a high-grade cancer, seminal vesicle invasion or lymph node metastases, (+) surgical margins had no effect on prognosis.
    - With extracapsular extension and a Gleason score ≤ 6, (+) surgical margins were associated with a higher progression rate.
    - Prognosis was adversely affected by (+) surgical margins only in moderately differentiated cancers with extracapsular extension alone.
    - If the cancer is otherwise confined, (+) surgical margins are associated with an excellent prognosis that is unlikely to be improved by adjuvant therapy.

- 93 patients who underwent radical prostatectomy and had seminal vesicle invasion without lymph node metastasis were evaluated.
  [Tefilli MV, J Urol **160**: 802–806, 1998]
  - Preoperative serum PSA, biopsy, and radical prostatectomy specimen Gleason score, surgical margin status, presence of extraprostatic extension, and evidence of biochemical disease progression were determined prospectively.
  - Biochemical failure was defined as a single serum PSA ↑ > 0.4 ng./ml.
  - RESULTS:
    - (+) surgical margins ($p = 0.001$), and Gleason score ≥ 7 from preoperative biopsies ($p = 0.03$) and from the radical prostatectomy specimens ($p = 0.01$) were significant predictors of disease progression at a median follow-up of 43.3 months.
    - ♂ with preoperative PSA <10 ng./ml → better DFS ($p = 0.07$).
    - On multivariate analysis, after adjusting for biopsy Gleason score, prostatectomy Gleason score, and serum PSA, (+) surgical margins remained a statistically significant predictor of disease progression ($p = 0.002$).

- Surgical margin status is an independent predictor of disease recurrence in patients with seminal vesicle involvement and (–) lymph nodes following radical prostatectomy.
- Serum PSA ≥ 10 ng/ml and specimen Gleason score ≥ 7 were also adverse prognostic factors in these patients.

Tumor ploidy and nuclear morphometry

[Adolfsson J, *Int J Cancer* **58**: 211–216, 1994]

- Results on correlating DNA ploidy with prognosis in prostate cancer are conflicting.

- Only half the studies published confirm ploidy to be an independent prognostic marker.

Histologic subtypes of cancer

- The recognition of histologic variants of prostate carcinoma is important because some types are associated with a different clinical outcome and might have a different therapeutic approach, and because awareness of the unusual pattern might be critical in avoiding diagnostic misinterpretations.

- 27 patients with small-cell anaplastic carcinoma of the prostate who presented to the Mayo Clinic from 1960 to 1990 were reviewed. [Oesterling JE, *J Urol* **147**: 804–807, 1992]

- Pathologically, small-cell anaplastic carcinoma of the prostate appears to be similar to oat-cell carcinoma of the lung.

- Small-cell anaplastic carcinoma of the prostate is highly malignant, is frequently of advanced stage at presentation, responds poorly to anti-androgen therapy, and has a poor prognosis.

Number of biopsies of the prostate

- It has been suggested that the best combination is to use PSA density, total PSA, and number of (+) biopsies. [Ackerman DA, *J Urol* **150**: 1845–1850, 1993]

- One study suggested that the best prediction is achieved by combining the Gleason score and the number of (+) biopsies. [Wills ML, *Urology* **51**: 759–764, 1998]

Molecular prognostic markers

[Katz AE, *Urology* **43**: 765–774, 1994]

- A number of studies have demonstrated the ability of the reverse transcription polymerase chain reaction (RT-PCR) to detect circulating prostate cells in patients with apparently localized disease undergoing radical prostatectomy.

- Other studies found a strong correlation between a (+) PCR reaction, capsular tumor penetration, and (+) surgical margins, suggesting the potential of this technique to be used for 'molecular staging' of prostate cancer.

- Attempts have been made to quantify mRNA for PSA in the blood stream of patients with clinically localized disease, and to make correlations with pathological staging.
  [Ylikoski A, *Eur Urol* **35**(Suppl 2): 97, 1999]

bcl-2

[Apakama I, *Br J Cancer* **74**: 1258–1262, 1996]
[Johnson MI, *Prostate* **37**: 223–229, 1998]

- *bcl-2* in the prostate is normally expressed in the basal epithelial cells, seminal vesicles, and ejaculatory ducts.

- In primary prostate cancer *bcl-2* is expressed in around 25% of cases.

- *bcl-2* overexpression is associated with increasing tumor stage and the development of hormone-refractory disease.

- *bcl-2* expression was highest in high-grade prostatic intraepithelial neoplasia vs benign prostatic hyperplasia and prostate cancer.

p53

[Apakama I, *Br J Cancer* **74**: 1258–1262, 1996]
[Moul JW, *Surgery* **120**: 159–166, 1996]

- *p53* positivity is absent in benign prostatic epithelium.

- *p53* nuclear positivity is present in about 20% of cases in primary prostate cancer.

- p53 protein accumulation appears to be a late event, and is associated with an advanced stage, a high Gleason tumor grade, hormone resistance, poor survival DNA aneuploidy, and a high cell proliferation rate.

- The combination of *bcl-2* overexpression and p53 nuclear protein accumulation in human prostate cancer has been shown to correlate with the development of hormone-refractory disease, and these are independent prognostic markers for recurrence post-radical prostatectomy.

pp32

[Visakorpi T, *Nature Med* **5**: 264–265, 1999]
[Kadkol SS, *Nature Med* **5**: 275–279, 1999]

- *pp32* is a nuclear phosphoprotein and tumor suppressor gene, which is expressed in nearly 90% of clinically significant prostate cancers.

- *pp32* expression is altered in prostate cancer, with benign prostatic tissue expressing *pp32* and carcinomas expressing the variants *pp32r1* and *pp32r2*.

Microvessel density

[Silberman MA, *Cancer* **79**: 772–779, 1997]

- ↑ Microvessel density correlates with ↑ Gleason score and the presence of metastases; it is an independent predictor of progression after radical prostatectomy for Gleason score 5–7 tumor.

Vascular endothelial growth factor

[Ferrer FA, *J Urol* **157**: 2329–2333, 1997]

- Expression is ↑ in prostate cancer compared with benign prostatic epithelium.

Perineural invasion

- 266 ♂ with $T_{1-3}N_XM_0$ prostate cancer and pretreatment PSA values < 10 ng/ml were treated with definitive external beam radiation therapy. [Anderson PR, *Int J Radiat Oncol Biol Phys* **41**: 1087–1092, 1998]

- RESULTS:
  - Univariate analysis according to pretreatment and treatment factors for biochemical no evidence of disease (bNED) control demonstrates a statistically significant improvement in 5-year bNED control for patients with Gleason score 2–6 vs 7–10, patients without evidence of perineural invasion vs those with perineural invasion, and patients with palpation stage T_1/T_{2ab} vs T_{2c}/T_3.
  - Multivariate analysis demonstrates that Gleason score ($p = 0.0496$), perineural invasion ($p = 0.0008$), and palpation stage ($p = 0.0153$) are significant independent predictors of bNED control.
- CONCLUSION:
  - This report identifies Gleason grades 7–10 and the presence of perineural invasion as well as palpation stage T_{2c}/T_3 as factors that predict worse bNED outcome for patients with a pretreatment PSA < 10 ng/ml who are treated with radiation therapy alone.

- 302 needle biopsies for perineural invasion for sensitivity and specificity in predicting capsular penetration in subsequent radical prostatectomies were evaluated.
  [Bastacky SI, *Am J Surg Pathol* **17**: 336–341, 1993]
  - RESULTS:
    - Perineural invasion was seen in 20% of needle biopsies, with a sensitivity of 27% and a specificity of 96% in predicting capsular penetration.
    - By including tumor with a Gleason sum ≥ 7 or perineural invasion on needle biopsy as being predictive, sensitivity ↑ to 36% with a specificity of 94%.
    - By restricting perineural invasion to cases with more than one nerve involved, or a nerve involvement of diameter ≥ 0.1 mm, specificity ↑ to 97% and 99%, respectively, with sensitivity ↓ to 15% and 9%, respectively.

- Actuarial bNED survival rates for 484 consecutive ♂ with clinically localized prostate carcinoma diagnosed by transrectal needle biopsy who completed three-dimensional conformal radiation therapy (3D CRT) alone.
  [Bonin SR, *Cancer* **79**: 75–80, 1997]
  - RESULTS:
    - The presence of perineural invasion predicted ↓ bNED survival in all patients. This detrimental effect, however, was confined to patients with pretreatment PSA values < 20 ng/ml.

- 349 previously untreated ♂ with prostatic adenocarcinoma who underwent bilateral pelvic lymphadenectomy and radical retropubic prostatectomy.
  [Egan AJ, *Am J Surg Pathol* **21**: 1496–1500, 1997]
  - All patients were clinically free of metastases and had cancer that was diagnosed on needle biopsy.
  - RESULTS:
    - Perineural invasion in needle biopsy of prostatic carcinoma has no independent predictive value for the presence of extraprostatic extension, seminal vesicle involvement, or pathologic stage in the radical prostatectomy.

- 80 radical prostatectomy cases that had perineural invasion on prostate needle biopsy were studied retrospectively to determine the presence and location of extraprostatic extension, (+) margins, and seminal vesicle or lymph node involvement, whether the neurovascular bundle had been excised, and whether tumor was present in the bundle region.
  [Holmes GF, *Urology* **53**: 752–756, 1999]
  - RESULTS:
    - When perineural invasion is seen on needle biopsy, the morbidity of resecting one or both neurovascular bundles, which in some cases could turn out to be unnecessary, must be weighed against the benefit of ↓ the incidence of (+) margins (17.5%) or ↓ the extent of (+) margins (11.3%).

- 212 ♂ with localized prostate cancer were evaluated for serum PSA, clinical stage, Gleason score, and the presence of perineural invasion.
  [Stone NN, *J Urol* **160**: 1722–1726, 1998]
  - RESULTS:
    - A (+) seminal vesicle biopsy is the most significant predictor of pelvic lymph node metastases in ♂ with T_1 or T_2 prostate cancer.
    - Perineural invasion is also an independent predictor of nodal disease.
    - Patients with either of these features should undergo pelvic lymph node dissection before receiving definitive therapy

- The significance of perineural invasion in prostate needle biopsy specimens for predicting extraprostatic extension is controversial.
  [Vargas SO, *Am J Clin Pathol* **111**: 223–228, 1999]
  - RESULTS:
    - In multivariate analysis, including preoperative serum PSA for 173 of the patients, the only independent predictor of extraprostatic extension was PSA.

- CONCLUSION:
  - While perineural invasion in biopsy specimens is a predictor of extraprostatic extension at resection that is independent of other histologic features, the positive predictive value is low and it is not an independent predictor when serum PSA is included.

Transforming growth factor-β1

[Byrne RL, *Br J Urol* **77**: 627–633, 1996]

- Transforming growth factor-β1 (TGF-β1) and TGF-β2 have been implicated in the development of prostatic disease.

- TGF-β1 has been detected immunohistochemically in both human prostatic stromal and epithelial cells.

- TGF-β2 mRNA has been identified in normal and malignant human prostate.

- The addition of TGF-β1 to cultured prostatic epithelial and stromal cells inhibits proliferation.

Bone morphogenetic proteins

[Hamdy FC, *Cancer Res* **57**: 4427–4431, 1997]
[Johnson M, *Eur Urol* **35**: 128, 1999]

- Bone morphogenetic protein-6 (BMP-6), in particular, is expressed in the majority of primary prostate cancers with established skeletal secondaries, and rarely in localized disease.

- Primary and secondary prostate cancer expresses BMP-6, which is found infrequently in skeletal metastases from other human malignancies.

- BMP-6 may have a role in the initiation of skeletal secondaries and the osteoblastic reaction commonly seen in these deposits.

- BMP-6 expression in primary prostate cancer was shown to have prognostic value in patients undergoing radical prostatectomy, predicting biochemical, clinical progression and ↓ survival.

Insulin-like growth factors

[Jones JI, *Endocrine Rev* **16**: 3–34, 1995]
[Kanety H, *J Clin Endocrin Metab* **77**: 229–233, 1993]

- Insulin-like growth factor-1 (IGF-1) and IGF-2 are important mitogens that mediate normal and neoplastic cell growth and bind to specific receptors, designated type I and II IGF receptors (IGFRs).

- IGFs are two of the most abundant growth factors in bone, the preferential site for metastatic prostate cancer.

- Type I IGFR is expressed by prostate cancer cells, which could facilitate the development of bone metastases.

- IGFs also have high affinity for a family of at least six IGF binding proteins (IGFBPs), which act to regulate their bioavailability.

- One study showed ↑ IGFBP-2 and ↓ IGFBP-3 in ♂ with prostate cancer.

Her-2/neu

[Craft N, *Nature Med* **5**: 280–285, 1999]

- Some studies have shown that *Her-2/neu* was overexpressed in a subset of prostate cancer patients, and serum levels of *Her2* extracellular domain have been correlated with hormone-refractory disease.

- Recent work suggests that *Her-2/neu* overexpression is involved with the emergence of hormone-resistant prostate cancer in vivo, by modulating the response of the androgen receptor to low doses of androgen.

Interleukin-6

[Waltregny D, *J Natl Cancer Inst* **90**: 1000–1008, 1998]

- Recent clinical studies have shown that elevated serum levels of interleukin-6 in prostate cancer patients correlate strongly with the presence of skeletal metastases.

Bone sialoprotein

[Waltregny D, *J Natl Cancer Inst* **90**: 1000–1008, 1998]

- Bone sialoprotein, a bone matrix protein, was found recently to be overexpressed in prostate cancer patients who demonstrate biochemical progression following treatment.

E-Cadherin

[Umbas R, *Cancer Res* **54**: 3929–3933, 1994]

- Immunocytochemistry performed on human prostate cancer samples showed a ↓ of E-cadherin expression in high-grade tumors, which is proving to be a powerful predictor of poor outcome, both in terms of disease progression and patient survival.

CD44

[Kallakury BVS, *Cancer* **78**: 1461–1469, 1996]

- CD44 is expressed on the plasma membrane of prostatic glandular cells. It is involved in cell adhesion as it acts as a receptor for the extracellular matrix components hyaluronic acid and osteopontin.

- In human prostate cancer CD44 down-regulation is correlated with high tumor grade, aneuploidy, and distant metastases.

Genetic factors

[Carter BS, *Proc Natl Acad Sci USA* **89**: 3367–3371, 1992]

- Hereditary prostate cancer, which can be separated from familial prostate cancer, has been reported to account for some 9% of all prostate cancer and > 40% of early onset disease.

Predictors of pathological stage before radical retropubic prostectomy

- The best predictors of pathological stage before radical retropubic prostectomy are combined paramenters.
  [Partin AW, *Urology* **58**: 843–848, 2001]

- The best validated are the Partin Tables, which provide the likelihood of various final pathological stages at radical retropubic prostatectomy.
  - Preoperative PSA.
  - Clinical (TNM) stage.
  - Biopsy Gleason score.

- These three variables were fitted using multinomial log–linear regression analysis to estimate the likelihood of organ-confined disease, extraprostatic extension, and seminal vesicle or lymph node status from the preoperative PSA.

Bone metabolic markers in advanced disease

- The most common marker of ↑ metabolic bone activity is serum alkaline phosphatase measurement.

- Bone alkaline phosphatase has been suggested to be a more sensitive and specific marker than total alkaline phosphatase.
  [Cooper EH, *Prostate* **25**: 236–240, 1994]

- Bone alkaline phosphatase was shown to enhance the clinical utility of PSA in staging prostate cancer, avoiding up to 32% of bone scans in detecting skeletal metastases.
  [Lorente JA, *Eur J Nucl Med* **26**: 625–632, 1999]

- The use of bone formation and resorption markers was assessed in a recent study using a combination of osteocalcin and bone alkaline phosphatase activity (bone formation), as well as deoxypyridinoline and pyridinoline cross-linked carboxy-terminal telopeptide of type I collagen (ICTP) (bone resorption).
  - Patients with and without evidence of skeletal metastases on bone scanning were studied.
  - RESULTS:
    - Levels of both sets of markers were ↑ and were as effective as bone scans in the detection of metastases.
    - ICTP was a better indicator of skeletal disease extent than was PSA.
    - Bone alkaline phosphatase was more sensitive than total alkaline phosphatase.
    - There was accelerated bone resorption evidenced by ↑ urinary hydroxyproline levels, bone histomorphometry, and radiological lytic appearance.
    [Maeda H, *J Urol* **157**: 539–543, 1997]

11

High-grade prostatic intraepithelial neoplasia

[Bostwick DG, *Mod Pathol* **17**(3): 360–379, 2004]
[Meng MV, *Urol Oncol* **21**(2): 145–151, 2003]

- High-grade prostatic intraepithelial neoplasia (HGPIN) is a precursor of prostate cancer.

- HGPIN pathologic criteria:
  - Intact basement membrane.
  - Enlarged, pleiomorphic nuclei.
  - Large, prominent nucleoli.

- HGPIN often coexists with prostate cancer.

- HGPIN is a very common pathologic finding in ♂, and the incidence ↑ with age.

- There is no strong correlation between HGPIN and prostatic-specific antigen (PSA).

- Finding prostate cancer on repeat biopsy after initial biopsy has demonstrated HGPIN is correlated with the number of initial biopsy cores obtained.
  - Repeat biopsy should be performed if the initial biopsy was a sextant (6 cores) biopsy or less.
  - Immediate repeat biopsy is not warranted for ♂ with HGPIN if the initial biopsy was an extended biopsy (≥ 10 cores).

HGPIN demonstrated during a sextant biopsy scheme should be repeated

- [Eggener SE, *J Urol* **174**(2): 500–504, 2005]
  - Retrospectively reviewed.
  - 24,893 ♂ enrolled in community prostate cancer screening.
  - Identified 1,202 ♂ with a PSA level of 2.6–4.0 ng/ml and a previous (–) biopsy.
  - *Caveat: ♂ typically only underwent sextant biopsy.*
  - RESULTS:
    - 136 ♂ eventually diagnosed with prostate cancer.
    - 106/136 (78%) underwent repeat biopsy for ↑ PSA.
    - 30/136 (22%) underwent repeat biopsy for ↑ PSA and suspicious digital rectal examination (DRE).
    - Of 48 ♂ with HGPIN on initial biopsy, 35% were subsequently diagnosed with prostate cancer compared to 12% without HGPIN on initial biopsy.
  - CONCLUSION:
    - ♂ with HGPIN on initial biopsy have a three-fold greater risk of subsequently being diagnosed with prostate cancer on a repeat biopsy compared to ♂ without HGPIN.

- [Borboroglu PG, *J Urol* **166**(3): 866–870, 2001]
  - Retrospective review.
  - 1,391 ♂ who underwent standard sextant biopsy (6 cores).
  - 137 (10%) ♂ had HGPIN or atypical small acinar proliferation (ASAP), 100 of whom underwent repeat biopsy within 12 months.
  - RESULTS:
    - 47/100 (47%) ♂ who underwent repeat biopsy within 1 year were found to have prostate cancer.
    - In only 22/47 (47%) ♂ was the cancer detected in the area of the initial HGPIN.
  - CONCLUSION:
    - Patients who undergo only sextant biopsy and have HGPIN are at ↑ risk of prostate cancer on repeat biopsy.

HGPIN demonstrated during an extended biopsy scheme does not warrant immediate repeat biopsy

- [Izawa JI, *BJU Int* **96**(3): 320–323, 2005]
  - 21 ♂ with HGPIN on initial prostate biopsy (mean: 7 cores) were reviewed retrospectively.

- All 21 ♂ had a repeat biopsy (mean: 8 cores) within 18 months of the initial biopsy.
- RESULTS:
  - 6/21 (29%) ♂ demonstrated prostate cancer on the second biopsy.
  - 3/21 (14%) ♂ demonstrated HGPIN on a second biopsy. All 3 ♂ had a third biopsy, but only 1 of 3 demonstrated prostate cancer.
  - 12/21 (57%) ♂ had a (–) second biopsy and were followed for a mean of 5 years. Five had a third (–) biopsy. None of these 12 developed clinically significant prostate cancer.
- CONCLUSIONS:
  - No patient with a (–) second or third prostate biopsy progressed to a diagnosis of clinically significant prostate cancer over more than 5 years of follow-up.
  - If a second sextant biopsy does not demonstrate prostate cancer, patients can be followed conservatively with PSA testing and DRE.

- [Lefkowitz GK, *Urology* **58**(6): 999–1003, 2001]
  - Retrospectively evaluated 103 ♂ with HGPIN demonstrated on a 12-core prostate biopsy.
  - 43/103 (42%) ♂ with HGPIN demonstrated on a 12-core biopsy underwent a second 12-core biopsy within 1 year of the initial biopsy.
  - RESULTS:
    - 1/43 (2.3%) of ♂ undergoing repeat 12-core biopsy within 1 year was found to have prostate cancer.
    - 20/43 (46.5%) ♂ had repeat HGPIN.
    - 20/43 (46.5%) ♂ had benign findings.
    - 1/43 (2.3%) ♂ had low-grade prostatic intraepithelial neoplasia.
    - 1/43 (2.3%) ♂ had atypia.
  - CONCLUSIONS:
    - A repeat biopsy after diagnosis of HGPIN on a 12-core biopsy rarely results in the detection of prostate cancer.
    - Immediate repeat biopsy (within 1 year) for HGPIN diagnosed on a 12-core biopsy is unnecessary.

- [Moore CK, *J Urol* **173**(1): 70–72, 2005]
  - 1,188 ♂ who had an initial extended prostate biopsy (≥ 10 cores) performed between January 1998 and February 2002.
  - Retrospectively reviewed 105/1,188 ♂ who had at least one repeat extended prostate biopsy secondary to the presence of HGPIN (33 ♂) or ASAP (72 ♂) on the initial extended prostate biopsy.
  - The time frame of the repeat extended biopsy was not stated.

- RESULTS:
  - Only 1/33 (3%) ♂ with a previous history of HGPIN on an extended prostate biopsy had prostate cancer on a repeat biopsy.
  - 11/33 ♂ with HGPIN in previous biopsies underwent a second repeated extended biopsy, and still none were diagnosed with prostate cancer.
  - 19/53 (36%) ♂ with a previous history of ASAP were found to have prostate cancer on repeat biopsy.
  - 3/19 (16%) of ♂ with ASAP who underwent a second extended biopsy were found to have prostate cancer.
- CONCLUSIONS:
  - HGPIN demonstrated in extended biopsies does not warrant a repeat biopsy.
  - ASAP, however, is associated with a risk of prostate cancer, and thus requires a second extended biopsy.

HGPIN and extended repeat biopsy at 3 years

- [Lefkowitz GK, J Urol **168**(4 Pt 1): 1415–1418, 2002]
  - Prospectively evaluated 31 ♂ with HGPIN demonstrated on an initial extended biopsy (12 cores) who underwent repeat extended biopsy 3 years later.
  - A single pathologist reviewed all biopsy specimens.
  - RESULTS:
    - 8/31 (26%) ♂ had prostate cancer on repeat biopsy at 3 years.
    - 11/31 (36%) ♂ had continued HGPIN.
    - 12/31 (39%) ♂ had benign findings.
    - The change in PSA was not significantly different between those with or without cancer on repeat biopsy.
  - CONCLUSIONS:
    - A high percentage of ♂ with HGPIN will develop prostate cancer 3 years after initial diagnosis.
    - These ♂ will develop prostate cancer independently of changes in PSA.
    - ♂ with HGPIN diagnosed on an extended prostate biopsy should undergo repeat biopsy 3 years after the initial diagnosis.

Relationship of HGPIN to prostate-specific antigen

- [Kim HL, Int Braz J Urol **28**(5): 413–416; discussion 417, 2002]
  - Retrospectively reviewed 61 cystoprostatectomy specimens from May 1992 to April 1999.

- These 61 ♂ had undergone cystoprostatectomy for bladder cancer without any known prostate pathology preoperatively.
- RESULTS:
  - 21/61 (34%) of prostate specimens demonstrated prostate cancer.
  - 46/61 (75%) of prostate specimens demonstrated HGPIN, including 21/21 (100%) with prostate cancer, and in 25/40 (63%) without prostate cancer.
  - Mean preoperative serum PSA in ♂ with HGPIN without prostate cancer was 1.9 ng/ml.
- CONCLUSIONS:
  - HGPIN is not an uncommon finding:
    - The incidence of HGPIN in ♂ undergoing cystoprostatectomy for bladder cancer → 63%.
  - HGPIN does not appear to elevate PSA.

Testosterone replacement in men with HGPIN

- [Rhoden EL, *J Urol* **170**(6 Pt 1): 2348–2351, 2003]
  - Retrospectively reviewed 75 hypogonadal ♂ who completed 12 months of testosterone replacement therapy (TRT).
  - All had biopsy (mostly sextant) on initiation of TRT.
  - 55/75 ♂ had a (–) biopsy.
  - 20/75 ♂ had HGPIN.
  - RESULTS:
    - PSA similar at baseline in ♂ with and without HGPIN.
    - PSA similar in both groups after 12 months of TRT.
    - 6 ♂ underwent repeat biopsy for ↑ PSA (4 in HGPIN (–) group and 2 in HGPIN (+) group): all (–).
    - 1 ♂ underwent repeated biopsy for abnormal DRE in HGPIN group: found to have prostate cancer.
  - CONCLUSION:
    - After 1 year of TRT ♂ with HGPIN do not have a greater ↑ in PSA or a significant risk of prostate cancer compared to ♂ without HGPIN.

12

External beam radiation therapy

[Pisansky TM, *N Engl J Med* **335**(15): 1583–1590, 2006]
[Speight JL, *J Clin Oncol* **23**(22): 8176–8185, 2005]
[Zelefsky MJ, *Int J Radiat Oncol Biol Phys* **53**(5): 1111–1116, 2002]

- Radical prostatectomy and radiation therapy were equally effective in appropriately selected patients with prostate cancer.
  [National Institutes of Health Consensus Development Panel, Consenus Statement: The Management of Clinically Localized Prostate Cancer, *NCI Monogr* **7**: 3–6, 1988]

Radiation therapy techniques

Conventional external beam techniques

- A simulator, a machine with identical isocentric gantry and table geometry as the treatment linear accelerator, is used to set up the patient position.

- The position of the normal structures and target is determined as follows:
  - The craniocaudal extent of the prostate is determined using an indwelling catheter with iodinated contrast in the balloon (for the cranial extent) and a retrograde urethrogram to localize the apex (approximately 0.5–1 cm above the contrast peak) (for the caudal extent).

- The anterior extent is posterior to the anterior cortex of the pubic symphysis.
- The posterior extent is anterior to the rectal wall (or S2/3 for whole pelvic fields).
- The rectal wall is visualized using either a contrast or a rectal catheter with radio-opaque markers.
- The patient is positioned and plain x-ray films of the treatment site are acquired.
- The films are marked to block normal structures and to indicate the treatment volume.
- The films are then used to fabricate customized blocks that block normal tissue and are mounted on the linear accelerator or treatment machine (or, alternatively, multileaf collimators may be used).
- A treatment plan is subsequently developed using a limited number of computerized tomography (CT) slices.
- Duplication of the position on the treatment table is achieved by lining up the skin tattoos to the lasers in the treatment room, which can define the isocentric geometry.

Limitations of conventional external beam radiation

- Only orthogonal fields (e.g. anteroposterior, right and left lateral, and posterior fields) or, occasionally, bilateral arcs can be used.

- High-energy beams (> 10 MVx) are needed to avoid an excessive dose to the subcutaneous tissues.

- A larger field or margin is needed to ensure coverage of the volume that needs to be treated.

- The treatment plan is seen on 1–3 CT scan slices, and these represent the entire treatment plan.
  - Thus, undesirable doses may be missed above or below the areas scanned.

- Errors related to the use of contrast may be introduced.
  - For example, retrograde urethrograms may lead to a systematic shift of the prostate in the superior direction, which may be > 5 mm in 23% of patients.
    [Malone S, *Int J Radiat Oncol Biol Phys* **46**: 89–93, 2000]
  - Furthermore, rectal barium (30 ml) may also result in a significant shift of the prostate ranging from −1.2 mm to +13.8 mm, which may result in a geographic miss.
    [Malone S, *Int J Radiat Oncol Biol Phys* **51**: 49–55, 2001]

Three-dimensional conformal and intensity modulated radiation therapy techniques

- The process begins with the acquisition of CT ± magnetic resonance imaging images and delineation of the treatment volume.
  - These CT volumetric images are used to plan the treatment.
  - In the case of intensity modulated radiation therapy (IMRT), inverse planning is done.

- Patient immobilization and position.
  - The prone position was previously thought to ↓ prostate mobility during treatment.
    [Zelefsky MJ, *Int J Radiat Oncol Biol Phys* **39**: 327–333, 1997]
  - However, recent data suggest that there is greater prostate motion during normal breathing in the prone, compared with the supine, position.
    [Dawson LA, *Int J Radiat Oncol Biol Phys* **48**: 319–323, 2000]
    [Malone S, *Int J Radiat Oncol Biol Phys* **48**: 105–109, 2000]

Treatment volume determination

- Treatment of the prostate alone.
  - The indication to include the prostate alone (i.e. to exclude the seminal vesicles from the treatment field) is low-risk disease (i.e. clinical T_{1c}–T_{2a} disease, Gleason score < 6, and prostate-specific antigen (PSA) < 10 ng/ml).
    [D'Amico A, *Int J Radiat Oncol Biol Phys* **39**: 335–340, 1997]
  - < 50% positive biopsies in low-risk disease has been suggested as a additional factor to be considered when deciding on treatments limited to the prostate alone.
    [Lieberfarb M, *Int J Radiat Oncol Biol Phys* **53**(4): 898–903, 2002]

- Treatment of the prostate and seminal vesicles.
  - If the risk of seminal vesicle involvement is > 15%, as calculated by one of the two validated methods:
    - The Roach formula: Risk of seminal vesicle involvement (%) = PSA + (Gleason score – 6) × 10
      [Roach M, *J Urol* **150**: 1923–1924, 1993]
      [Roach M 3rd, *Int J Radiat Oncol Biol Phys* **28**(1): 33–37, 1994]
    - Partin's tables: these give the percentage risk of seminal vesicle involvement based on the T stage, Gleason score, and PSA.
      [Partin A, *Urology* **58**(6): 843–848, 2001]
      [Augustin H, *J Urol* **171**: 177–181, 2004]

- Treatment of the whole pelvis.
  [Roberts T, *Semin Radiat Oncol* **13**(2): 109–120, 2003]
  - Pelvic radiation is recommended.
    - When pelvic lymph node risk is > 15% by Partin's tables, or there is > 15% risk of positive pelvic nodes by the Roach formula.
      [Roach M, *Int J Radiat Oncol Biol Phys* **28**(1): 33–37, 1994]
    - Patients with suspicious pelvic nodes on CT.
  - Target volume: prostate and periprostatic tissue, seminal vesicles, obturator node, internal iliac nodes, external iliac nodes, and presacral nodes (which are situated anterior to anterior to S1–S2 sacral segments).
  - Field arrangement: four-field box technique (AP, PA, RT LAT, LT LAT); the superior border is at the L5/S1 interspace (for a mini-pelvic field, the superior border is at the midsacrum); the inferior border is 1 cm distal to the apex on the urethrogram, usually at or below the bottom of the ischial tuberosities; laterally, the borders are 1.5–2.0 cm lateral to the pelvic inlet, and anteriorly the border is at the anterior cortex of the pubic symphysis; the posterior border is at the inferior aspect of the midportion of the S3 segment or S2/3.
  - More recently, IMRT and three-dimensional conformal techniques have been described for the treatment of pelvic nodes.
    [Ashman J, *Int J Radiat Oncol Biol Phys* **63**(3): 765–771, 2005].
  - Dose: 45–46 Gy in 1.8–2 Gy fractions over 4.5–5 weeks.

Results of studies of treatment volume determination

Pelvic vs prostate radiation in the PSA era

- **Radiation Therapy Oncology Group (RTOG) 94–13.**
  [Roach M, *Proc ASTRO* **51**(Suppl 1): 3, 2001]
  [Lawton C, *Proc ASTRO* **63**(Suppl 1): S19, 2005]
  - 1,323 ♂ with clinically localized prostate cancer, PSA < 100 ng/ml, and an estimated lymph node risk > 15% (by Roach formula).
  - Prospective, randomized trial to determine the optimum timing of hormone therapy (flutamide 250 mg p.o. t.i.d. and leuprolide or goserelin), and to determine the optimum extent of radiation field.
  - Group I: prostate radiation and neoadjuvant hormone therapy given 2 months prior to radiation + 2 months with radiation (PO RT + NHT).
  - Group II: prostate radiation and adjuvant hormone therapy given 4 months after completing radiation (PO RT + AHT).

- Group III: pelvic radiation and neoadjuvant hormone therapy given 2 months prior to radiation + 2 months with radiation (WP RT + NHT).
- Group IV: pelvic radiation and adjuvant hormone therapy given 4 months after completing radiation (WP RT + AHT).
- Median follow-up → 5.9 years.
- RESULTS:

	PO RT + NHT (n = 324)	PO RT + AHT (n = 323)	WP RT NHT (n = 325)	WP RT + AHT (n = 323)
5-year progression-free survival rate	36.8%	40.4%	48.3%	38.1%
5-year biochemical failure	45.5%	40%	35.9%	42.8%

- – WP RT + NHT had a significantly improved progression-free survival over PO RT + NHT ($p = 0.0041$) and WP RT + AHT ($p = 0.0045$).
- – A marginal improvement was seen as compared with WP RT + AHT ($p = 0.0656$).
- – WP RT + NHT had a significantly improved biochemical failure compared with PO RT + NHT ($p = 0.0070$) and marginal improvement compared with WP RT + AHT ($p = 0.0699$).

- Prostate and seminal vesicle radiation vs prostate radiation alone. [Lieberfarb M, *Int J Radiat Oncol Biol Phys* **51**: 114–115, 2001]
  - 2,099 ♂ with clinically localized prostate cancer underwent radical retropubic prostatectomy (RRP).
  - Retrospective study.
  - Median follow-up → 44 months.
  - Primary endpoints:
    - – Pathologic seminal vesicle invasion (SVI).
    - – Extracapsular extension (ECE) ± positive margins.
    - – 5-year postoperative PSA outcome.
  - RESULTS:
    - – Patients in the low-risk category (PSA < 10 ng/ml, ≤ T_{2a} and Gleason 2–6) with ≤ 50% (+) needle biopsies, and intermediate-risk patients (T_{2b} *or* Gleason 7 *or* PSA > 10 ng/ml but < 20 ng/ml) with ≤ 17% (+) needle biopsies, have very low

risk of SVI (2–3%) or ECE (7–9% if margins (–) and 4–11% if margins (+)), and ≥ 90–93% PSA failure-free survival.
- Thus, these patients were optimal candidates for prostate-only radiation, with exclusion of the seminal vesicles from the treatment field.

- Whole vs partial seminal vesicle radiation.
  [Kestin L, *Proc ASTRO* **51**: 138, 2001]
  - Specimens from 268 ♂ undergoing prostatectomy were reviewed by a designated pathologist.
  - 60 specimens showed seminal vesicle invasion (SVI).
  - RESULTS:
    - Factors influencing seminal vesicle invasion included:
      - The presence of disease bilaterally within the prostate (18% vs 2% SVI).
      - The presence of (+) margins (30% vs 4% SVI).
      - The presence of (+) nodes (56% vs 14% SVI).
    - Factors found to predict SVI on multivariate analysis:
      - Higher percentage of the gland involved by the tumor.
      - Maximum tumor size within the gland.
      - Gleason score.
      - The presence or absence of extracapsular extension.
      - When SVI occurred, the median length of involvement was 1 cm (90th percentile: 2 cm).
    - Since the median seminal vesicle length was 4 cm it was concluded that radiation therapy can be limited to the proximal half of the gland.
    - This is an option for intermediate-risk disease.
    - We do <u>not</u> recommend this in high-risk disease.

- Dose and gross tumor volume prescription.
  - The International Committee on Radiation Units and Measurements (ICRU) published guidelines for reporting, recording, and prescribing radiation doses. It was recommended that a reference point, and minimum and maximum doses be reported. The ICRU reference point should be a point within the target, usually close to the isocenter of the beams. There should be a 3–7% heterogeneity between the minimum and the isocenter dose.
    [ICRU, *Prescribing, Reporting, and Recording Photon Beam Therapy*, ICRU, Bethesda, MD, 1993]
  - For conformal treatment, the gross tumor volume must include the whole prostate for stage T_1–T_{2a} disease, and the prostate and seminal vesicles for stage T_{2b} disease, and also include any extraprostatic

extension in patients with T_3 tumors. The planned target volume is 0.7–0.8 cm around the prostate or seminal vesicles or peri-prostatic tumor. Non-uniform smaller margins are used posteriorly over the rectum. An additional 0.6 cm margin from the planning target volume (PTV) to the block edge should be added to account for penumbra; internal motion is a concern and varies in the range 4–8 mm for the prostate and 7–11 mm for the seminal vesicles.

Radiation therapy dose–response

[Zeitman A, JAMA **294**(10): 1233–1239, 2005]
[Kupelian P, Int J Radiat Oncol Biol Phys **61**(2): 415–419, 2005]

- Results obtained using 70 Gy of conventional external beam radiation therapy ALONE for locally advanced disease $(T_{2c}-T_4)$.
  - 30–50% develop a palpable local recurrence within 10 years, and the majority will develop distant metastases.
    [Hanks GE, Int J Radiat Oncol Biol Phys **27**: 125–127, 1993]
  - Thus, dose escalation is needed.

Studies of dose escalation

- [Zeitman A, JAMA **294**(10): 1233–1239, 2005]
  - 393 patients with $T_{1b}-T_{2b}$ cancer and PSA < 15 ng/ml.
  - Prospective randomized trial of two doses of proton external beam radiation.
    - Group I: 70.2 Gy.
    - Group II: 79.2 Gy.
  - Median follow-up: 5.5 years.
  - Main outcome measure: freedom from biochemical failure at 5 years.
  - RESULTS: 5-year freedom from biochemical failure*

	Whole group (n = 393)	High- and intermediate-risk group (n = 162)	Low-risk group (n = 227)
Group I: conventional dose (70.2 Gy)	61.4%	63.4%	60.1%
Group II: high dose (79.2 Gy)	80.4%	79.5%	80.5%
	$p = 0.001$	$p = 0.03$	$p < 0.001$

*One patient refused to participate after randomization, and 3 patients were not classified by risk status.

- [Pollack A, *Int J Radiat Oncol Biol Phys* **53**: 1097–1105, 2002]
  - 301 patients.
  - Prospective, randomized, dose-escalation trial (no androgen deprivation allowed).
  - Clinical stage $T_{1-3}N_XM_0$ prostate cancer treated between 1993 and 1998.
  - Randomized to two groups:
    - Group I: 70 Gy (150 patients).
    - Group II: 78 Gy (151 patients).
  - Median follow-up → 5 years.
  - RESULTS:
    - Increasing the dose from 70 Gy to 78 Gy to isocenter led to a higher 5-year freedom from failure (FFF), including a biochemical failure of 64% vs 70% ($p = 0.03$).
    - In patients with a PSA > 10 ng/ml, dose escalation significantly improved FFF to 62% for the 78 Gy group vs 43% for the 70 Gy group; and led to a higher freedom from distant metastases of 98% vs 88% at 6 years ($p = 0.056$) for the 78 Gy group.
    - Dose escalation did <u>not</u> show a difference in patients with stage cT_1–T_2 and PSA < 10 ng/ml.

- [Kupelian P, *Int J Radiat Oncol Biol Phys* **61**(2): 415–419, 2005]
  - 4,839 patients.
  - Retrospective combined data from nine institutions.
  - Group I: dose < 72 Gy.
  - Group II: dose > 72 Gy.
  - Endpoint: 5-year PSA disease-free survival.
  - Median follow-up → 5.8 and 5.7 years for groups I and II, respectively.
  - RESULTS:
    - Dose was an independent factor affecting 5-year PSA disease-free survival ($p < 0.001$).

- [Zelefsky M, *Int J Radiat Oncol Biol Phys* **41**: 491–500, 1998]
  - 743 patients with clinically localized prostate cancer (T_{1c}–T_3).
  - Treated between 1988 and 1995.
  - Phase I, dose-escalation study of three-dimensional conformal radiation therapy (3D-CRT) of doses as follows:
    - 64.8, 70.2y, 75.6, and 81 Gy to the isodose line covering the volume to be treated.
    - In the 81 Gy group the rectum was completely blocked after 72 Gy.
  - Median follow-up → 3 years.

- RESULTS:
  - Dose escalation in favorable risk patients did not significantly impact PSA outcome.
  - Dose escalation to > 75.6 Gy improved local control and PSA relapse-free survival in intermediate (53% vs 79%; $p = 0.04$) and unfavorable risk groups (33% vs 59%; $p = 0.03$).
  - A significant ↑ in the percentage of (–) biopsies with increased dose was seen, from 30% in the 66.6 Gy group to 53% in the 81 Gy group.

- [Pinover WH, *Int J Radiat Oncol Biol Phys* **47**: 649–454, 2000]
  - 488 patients with prostate cancer (clinical stage T_{1-3}, Gleason score 2–10, PSA < 10 ng/ml) were treated with three-dimensional conformal radiation therapy (3D-CRT) alone between 1989 and 1997.
  - Prospective dose-escalation trial.
  - Radiation: total dose = 63–79 Gy.
  - Median follow-up → 3 years.
  - Analysis was by prognostic group.
    - The poor prognostic group had cT_{2b}–T_3, or Gleason score > 7, or perineural invasion.
    - The good prognostic group had none of these factors.
  - Endpoint = biochemical no evidence of disease (NED) rate by American Society for Therapeutic Radiology and Oncology (ASTRO) definition.
  - RESULTS:
    - The 5-year biochemical NED rates were 70%, 75% and 94% for radiation doses of < 72.5, 72.5–75.99, and ≥ 76 Gy, respectively ($p = 0.006$) in patients with the additional risk factors of cT_{2b}–T_3, Gleason score > 7, or perineural invasion.
    - No significant differences were seen in the remaining patients who did not have these poor prognosticators.
    - Radiation therapy dose escalation to ≥ 76 Gy with 3D-CRT improves the 5-year biochemical NED rate for patients with localized prostate cancer with stage, even if their PSA is < 10 ng/ml. (*Note*: these patients did not receive hormone-deprivation therapy.)

- RTOG 9406.
  [Ryu JK, *Int J Radiat Oncol Biol Phys* **54**(4): 1036–1046, 2002]
  - Dose-escalation study: 68.4 Gy in 1.8 Gy fractions to 78 Gy in 2 Gy fractions.
  - Eligibility criteria: all N_0M_0 prostate cancer with PSA < 70 ng/ml except stage T_{1a}, T_{1b}–T_{2b} with Gleason score 2–5 and PSA < 4 ng/ml, or T_4; Karnofsky performance status (KPS) > 80.

- Stratification by prognostic group:
  - Group I: cT_{1b}–T_{2b} with ≤ 15% risk of seminal vesicle involvement (calculated using Roach formula).
  - Group II: cT_{1b}–T_{2b} with > 15% risk of seminal vesicle involvement (calculated using Roach formula), and cT_{2c} with PSA < 70 ng/ml.
  - Group III: cT_3 with PSA < 70 ng/ml.
- Only toxicity data available.

Treatment recommendation

- Doses > 72 Gy reduce the risk of PSA failure in patients with intermediate- to high-risk disease and, more recently, even in low-risk disease.

- Whole-pelvis radiation should be considered if the risk of pelvic lymph node positivity is ≥ 15%.

13

Pelvic node radiation in prostate cancer

Introduction and background: how commonly are lymph nodes involved?

- The role of pelvic lymph node (LN) irradiation in the treatment of clinically localized prostate cancer continues to be controversial.

- Recent data suggest the incidence of LN involvement is > previously thought.
  - Most estimates are based on patients who underwent an incomplete node dissection.
  - Even LNs that were removed and considered (–) by standard cytological evaluation may be involved if more sensitive tests are performed.

- Treatment of pelvic LNs either surgically or by radiation may be beneficial.
  - This body of literature when taken as a whole suggests that:
    - It is important to identify patients with occult LN involvement.
    - Treatment of these nodes is beneficial.
    - External beam radiotherapy (EBRT) in combination with neoadjuvant hormone therapy may be the ideal approach for comprehensively addressing occult nodal disease.

Nomograms and algorithms for estimating the risk of LN involvement

- When LN invasion is documented pathologically, some surgeons favor aborting radical prostatectomy and initiate either immediate or

delayed hormone therapy, while others complete the intended operation with subsequent androgen ablation.
- This latter approach potentially prolongs time to recurrence and ↑ cancer specific survival.

- Pelvic LN dissection (PLND) could play a role in either case, as a staging modality or potentially as a therapeutic intervention.

- There is controversy surrounding the indications for PLND because of the need to balance the low prevalence of LN metastasis in low-stage patients against the morbidity and treatment cost.
  - Thus PLND is not routinely recommended.

- In order to define patients who do not need to go through a PLND, several nomograms have been derived, primarily to avoid lymphadenectomy in low-risk patients.

- Retrospective, non-randomized analysis of 5,510 patients with complete clinical and pathological information treated with radical prostatectomy at six institutions between 1985 and 2000.
  [Cagiannos I, *J Urol* **70**: 1798–1803, 2003]
  - The major exclusion criteria included prior hormone therapy, and pretreatment PSA > 50 ng/ml.
  - LN metastases were detected in 206 (3.7%) patients.
  - The authors recommended omitting PLND when their nomogram predicts a probability of ≤ 1.5–3% LN involvement.
  - In this study 'standard template pelvic LNs dissection' was performed.
  - An extended PLND (ELND) and the use of more sensitive technologies (other than simple light microscopy) would be expected to yield a substantially higher incidence of LN involvement.
  - The threshold proposed in this study: patients with a Gleason score of 7 and a PSA ~ 8 ng/ml are at a significant risk of LN involvement.

- Using the so-called 'Roach LN equation', such a patient would also be considered appropriate for pelvic radiotherapy (RT).
  [Roach M, *J Urol* **150**: 1923–1924, 1993]

- The Hamburg algorithm categorizes patients into three risk groups for LN metastasis.
  [Haese A, *Cancer* **95**: 1016–1021, 2002]
  - All patients with ≥ 4 of 6 biopsies containing any Gleason pattern 4 are considered 'high risk', and patients with ≥ 1 of 6 biopsies containing dominant Gleason pattern 4 are categorized as inter-

mediate risk, predicting likelihoods of LN metastasis of 45% and 19%, respectively.
- All other patients make up the low-risk group, with a likelihood of metastasis of 2.2%, and ELND is <u>not</u> indicated for these patients.

Extended lymphadenectomy: increased detection and therapeutic benefit?

- ELND may substantially ↑ the detection of LN metastasis compared to a standard dissection.

- Recent studies have shown that there is a high rate of LN metastasis outside of the fields of standard lymphadenectomy in patients with clinically localized prostate cancer.
[Heidenreich A, J Urol **167**: 1681–1686, 2002]
  - It is recommended that ELND only be performed in patients with a high risk of LN involvement (PSA > 10.5, Gleason sum ≥ 7), and omitted in the low-risk group of patients.

- In addition to an ↑ detection rate, there may also be a significant benefit in biochemical recurrence-free survival for certain subgroups undergoing ELND.
[Allaf ME, J Urol **172**: 1840–1844, 2004]

- Patients who undergo a more extensive lymphadenectomy may have ↓ long-term risk of prostate-cancer-related death.
  - Even in patients with (–) LNs compared with patients without lymphadenectomy.
[Joslyn SA, Urology **68**: 121–125, 2006]

ELND in patients with PSA < 10 ng/ml: is it really necessary?

- Controversy persists concerning the role of PLND in patients with a preoperative PSA < 10 ng/ml.

- (+) LNs in ~ 11% of patients with a PSA < 10 ng/ml.
[Schumacher MC, Eur Urol **50**: 272–279, 2006]
  - It is recommended that the number of LNs removed with ELND is in the range 18–28, compared with 9–11 LNs for a limited LN dissection.
  - (+) LNs were found along the internal iliac vessels in 73% of patients, either exclusively or in combination with another area.

- Incidence of LN metastasis is low in patients with a PSA < 10 ng/ml and a Gleason score ≤ 6.
  - In these patients ELND may not be necessary.
- For the high-risk group, with a Gleason score ≥ 7, despite a PSA < 10 ng/ml, ELND is mandatory.

- Of the preoperative predictors of LN involvement, PSA is the weakest, with several studies indicating that even with low PSA values the risk of LN invasion is non-negligible.
  [Stamey TA, J Urol **172**: 1297–1301, 2004]

Patients who are pathologically node negative

Locally advanced node-negative prostate cancer

[Pagliarulo V, J Clin Oncol **24**: 2735–2742, 2006]

- The studies reviewed above all assumed that the gold standard for detecting LN involvement was standard cytopathologic evaluation.

- Some studies suggest that either more careful sectioning of the LNs, or the application of the reverse transcriptase polymerase chain reaction (RT-PCR), or PSA n-RNA copy number might allow the identification of cancer in nodes otherwise considered N_0.

- Patients with extraprostatic tumor extension (stage T_3) are at ↑ risk for progression, even in the absence of histopathologic evidence of LN metastasis.
  [Partin AW, JAMA **277**: 1445–1451, 1997]

- Investigators from the University of Southern California used immunohistochemical assessment of LNs to detect tumors not recognized at initial histologic examination.
  - They found occult LN metastasis in 13% of patients with pT_3N_0 prostate cancer that was associated with a significantly ↑ risk of recurrence and death.

- Investigators from Baylor University described the RT-PCR as a more sensitive method than histology for detecting small numbers of disseminated cells.
  [Shariat SF, J Clin Oncol **21**: 1223–1231, 2003]
  - They noted that, overall, 20% of N_0 patients had evidence of involvement using this assay.
  - They used a highly sensitive and specific RT-PCR assay for human glandular kallikrein 2 (hK2) mRNA to differentially amplify splice variants of the *hKLK2* gene.

- They noted that RT-PCR/hK2 was strongly associated with progression, failure, development of metastases, and prostate-cancer-specific mortality.

- Similarly investigators from Mt Sinai reported they could correlate the risk of subsequent progression by measuring, the PSA mRNA copies in N_0 pelvic lymph node (PLN) patients.
  [Ferrari AC, *J Clin Oncol* **24**: 3081–3088, 2006]
  - They noted that normalized PSA copies (PSA-N) $\geq$ 100 was an independent molecular criterion for identifying high-risk patients with occult micrometastasis but N_0 by standard cytopathologic evaluation.

Can imaging improve the detection of lymph node metastasis?

Role of sentinel lymph node dissection

- Study suggests that there may be a role for combining preoperative prostate lymphoscintigraphy with intraoperative radio-guided surgery to identify sentinel lymph node (SLN) involvement in patients with clinically localized prostate cancer.
  - Radio-guided surgery by transrectally applying technetium-99m nanocolloid under ultrasonographic guidance 1 day before lymphadenectomy directly into the prostate.
  - Two hours after the injection, scintigrams were taken and the individual location of the SLN identified.
  - > half of the patients have (+) LNs outside the region of a standard LN.

Magnetic resonance imaging based nanoparticle detection of occult LN metastasis in prostate cancer

- Although magnetic resonance imaging (MRI) based imaging provides excellent anatomical detail and soft tissue contrast, it has been shown to be suboptimal for routine application in the detection of nodal metastasis.
  [Forman JD, *Radiology* **215**(Suppl): 1373–1382, 2000]

- Studies have shown that by adding lymphotropic superparamagnetic nanoparticles containing densely packed dextrans the sensitivity of MRI can be dramatically improved.
  - Using this agent combined with high-resolution MRI, small and otherwise undetectable LN metastasis in patients with prostate

cancer can be identified and selectively targeted.
[Harisinghani MG, *N Engl J Med* **348**: 2491–2499, 2003]
- Technical difficulties and a lack of US Food and Drug Adminis-tration approval have hampered the widespread adoption of this technology.
- However, with standardization of criteria for defining abnormal studies, it is likely that this technology will prove useful for design-ing EBRT fields in the future.
[Harisinghani MG, *Am J Roentgenol* **186**: 144–148, 2006]

Treatment of patients with pelvic lymph nodes: a role for radiotherapy?

Hormone therapy (HT), EBRT + HT, and EBRT alone

- Experts do not agree on what is the most appropriate treatment for patients with metastatic spread to pelvic LNs.

- Several trials suggest that immediate HT should be considered instead of deferred treatment started at clinical progression for patients with spread to regional LNs.

- Immediate adjuvant HT after definitive local procedure (radical pros-tatectomy with pelvic lymphadenectomy or radiation) may ↓ pro-gression rates and improve survival in patients with LN (+) prostate cancer.
[Messing EM, *Int J Radiat Oncol Biol Phys* **44**: 801–808, 1999]

- Numerous studies have shown that there is a favorable interaction between HT and irradiation.
- The addition of EBRT may improve the outcomes compared to HT alone.
[Roach M, *J Urol* **170**: S35–S40; discussion S40–S31, 2003]

Prophylactic irradiation for LNs

- Occult LN involvement despite negative imaging is a well-recognized problem in patients with prostate cancer.

- Danish Breast Cancer Cooperative Group 82c (DBCG 82c).
[Overgaard M, *Lancet* **353**: 1641–1648, 1999]
- Prophylactic nodal RT has been shown to prolong survival in a large randomized trial of ♀ with breast cancer.

- What is the role of prophylactic pelvic LN irradiation in intermediate- to high-risk prostate cancer patients?
  - Because a higher risk of complications and a higher cost might be expected with the addition of whole-pelvic radiotherapy (WPRT), it would be desirable to omit this treatment if it were not beneficial.

- Radiation Therapy Oncology Group (RTOG) 77–06.
  [Asbell SO, *Int J Radiat Oncol Biol Phys* **15**: 1307–1316, 1988]
  - A prospective randomized trial.
  - Failed to demonstrate a benefit with WP RT.
  - LIMITATION OF THE STUDY:
    - Included patients estimated to be at low risk of LN involvement, pathologically LN (–) (or by imaging) and PSA was not used.

- RTOG 9413.
  [Roach M, *J Clin Oncol* **21**: 1904–1911, 2003]
  - Data indicate that patients with a risk of LN involvement of > 15% might benefit from prophylactic WP RT.
  - The only modern randomized trial addressing this issue demonstrated that WP RT + neoadjuvant and concurrent hormone therapy (NHT) is associated with a significantly longer freedom from progression compared with prostate-only radiotherapy (PO RT) + NHT, PO RT + adjuvant hormone therapy (AHT) and WP RT + AHT in patients with a risk of LN involvement of > 15%.
  - In a subset analysis, patients with a risk of LN involvement of 15–35% benefited the most from pelvic nodal RT, whereas those with a risk of < 15% or > 35% benefit less from pelvic node RT.
    - Thus some patients may not benefit because their risk is too low, whereas others may not benefit because their risk of systemic disease is too high.
  - The study reached its primary endpoint, demonstrating an improvement in progression-free survival (PFS) with the addition of WP RT.
  - CONCLUSION:
    - In the absence of a larger, more compelling, randomized trial, these data suggest that RTOG 9413 established NHT + WP RT as the standard of care in patients with intermediate- to high-risk disease.

- Some retrospective studies suggest that there is no benefit from the addition of HT and WP RT to patients with a risk of nodal involvement > 15%.
  [Jacob R, *Int J Radiat Oncol Biol Phys* **61**: 695–701, 2005]
  - However, selection bias, small sample size, failure to consistently

use NHT in all patients, and suboptimal field size can easily explain such findings.
[Roach M, *Int J Radiat Oncol Biol Phys* **66**: 647–653, 2006]
- The optimum benefit of WP RT appears to require the use of neoadjuvant HT and comprehensive WP RT.

- RTOG 85–31.
  [Pilepich MV, *Int J Radiat Oncol Biol Phys* **61**: 1285–1290, 2005]
  - Patients with advanced disease (Gleason score > 6, T_3, and PSA > 30 ng/ml) appear to benefit from the use of long-term AHT in addition to WP RT.

- Intensity modulated radiotherapy.
  - With the availability of sophisticated computerized planning systems, one should consider full-dose RT for local control of prostate tumors with spread to local LNs but without distant metastasis.

- Intensity-modulated radiotherapy improves pelvic LN coverage without the cost of greatly increasing the dose and coverage to critical structures such as the bladder, rectum, small bowel, and penile bulb.
  [A. Wang-Cheseboro, *Int J Radiat Oncol Biol Phys* **66**: 654–662, 2006]

Conclusions

- The incidence of pelvic LNs by metastasis in ♂ with clinically localized prostate cancer is significantly greater than commonly believed.

- Most studies are based on inadequate nodal sampling and fail to use the most sensitive approaches for identifying disease in the LNs.

- Hormone therapy combined with intensity-modulated radiotherapy represents an ideal strategy for addressing occult nodal disease, even in the most difficult places.
  [Murray SK, *Am J Surg Pathol* **28**: 1154–1162, 2004]

Selected papers on the incidence of pelvic lymph node involvement (2006)

See Table 13.1 on the following pages.

Table 13.1 The incidence of pelvic lymph node involvement: selected studies

Study	Methodology	Key findings
[Joslyn SA, *Urology* 68: 121–125, 2006]	Data on all patients undergoing radical prostatectomy for prostate cancer obtained from the SEER Program (1988–1991). All surviving patients had a minimum follow-up of 10 years. Of 57,764 ♂, 13,020 (22.5%) underwent radical prostatectomy. The median survival time was 127 months. Most tumors were diagnosed as localized stage and SEER grade 2 (Gleason score 5 or 6; Gleason pattern 3, moderately differentiated)	A relationship was noted between the number of LNs removed and examined at prostatectomy for prostate cancer and the likelihood of finding LN metastasis and an ↑ in the prostate-cancer-specific survival, even in patients who had histologically (–) LNs. Patients with > 1 (+) LN had a significantly greater risk of prostate-cancer-related death
[Schumacher MC, *Eur Urol* 50: 272–279, 2006]	Patients with localized prostate cancer and PSA < 10 ng/ml with (–) staging examinations who underwent radical prostatectomy with bilateral ELND and ≥ 10 LNs. (*n* = 231) and median PSA 6.7 ng/ml	(+) LNs were found in 11%; the majority (25%) had a Gleason score ≥ 7, whereas only 3% were node (+) with a Gleason score ≤ 6. (+) LNs were found in the internal iliac vessels in 73%, either exclusively or in combination with another area

Continued

Continued

Table 13.1   *Continued*

Study	Methodology	Key findings
[Pagliarulo V, *J Clin Oncol* **24**: 2735–2742, 2006]	274 patients with pT_3 prostate cancer treated by radical prostatectomy and bilateral LN dissection. 180 were staged N_0, while 94 were LN(+). LNs from the 180 patients were evaluated for occult metastasis by immunohistochemistry. Recurrence and overall survival were compared among patients with occult tumor cells (OTN(+)), with patients whose LNs remain negative (OLN(–)) and with the 94 LN (+) patients	Occult tumor cells were found in 24/180 (13.3%) N_0 patients. OLN(+) was significantly associated with ↑ recurrence and ↓ survival compared with OLN(–) patients. Outcome for patients with OLN(+) disease was similar to that for patients with LN(+) disease. The authors concluded that the use immunohistochemistry can allow detection of tumors not recognized at initial histology, identifying patients who might benefit from early administration of adjuvant systemic treatment
[Ferrari AC, *J Clin Oncol* **24**: 3081–3088, 2006]	Quantitative measures of PSA mRNA copies in N_0 PLN, defined by PSA-N, and a threshold PSA-N $\geq$ 100 vs PSA-N < 100 copies, were assessed by continuous and categorical multivariate analyses to be independent	The 4-year, biochemical-failure-free survival of patients with PSA-N $\geq$ 100 vs < 100 was 55% and 77% ($p < 0.05$). PSA-N identify occult mets in N_0 PLN. PSA-N $\geq$ 100 is a new, independent molecular staging criterion for localized prostate cancer that identifies high-risk patients with clinically significant but occult micrometastasis

Continued

Table 13.1 *Continued*		
Study	**Methodology**	**Key findings**
[Weckermann D, *Br J Urol Int* **97**: 1173–1178, 2006]	414 patients with PSA ≤ 10 ng/ml and a biopsy Gleason score of ≤ 6 and (+) biopsies in one (group 1) or both (group 2) lobes	In > 50% nodes were outside STD nodal region. The authors concluded that, when performing PLND, extended or radio-guided surgery should be preferred, as > half of patients have (+) LNs outside the region of a standard LN
[Granfors T, *J Urol* **176**: 544–547, 2006]	91 patients with newly diagnosed prostate cancer randomized after LN staging to receive EBRT or combined orchiectomy and EBRT (45). Follow-up > 14 years	87% of patients in the EBRT group and 76% in the combined orchiectomy and EBRT group died. Prostate cancer mortality was 57% and 36%, respectively, favoring combined treatment, with benefit mainly seen in LN (+) tumors

SEER, Surveillance, Epidemiology, and End Results.

14

Prostate brachytherapy

Low dose rate brachytherapy

[Zietman AL, *Curr Treat Options Oncol* **3**(5): 429–436, 2002]
[Blasko JC, *Semin Radiat Oncol* **12**(1): 81–94, 2002]

- Brachytherapy ('close' therapy) is the placement of radioactive sources into or near tumors for therapeutic purposes.

- Permanent interstitial implantation was initially reported in 1913, when the temporary placement of radium-containing needles into the prostate through a urethral catheter was described.
  [Pasteau D, *Arch Roentgenol Ray* **28**: 396, 1913]
  – Due to radiation safety issues and the numerous complications seen, this technique was eventually replaced.

- In the 1920s, researchers at the Johns Hopkins Hospital performed the first transperineal implants of radium needles into the prostate in the USA.
  [Young H, *Surg Gynecol Obstet* **34**: 93–98, 1922]

- This was followed by permanent brachytherapy using radioactive gold (^{198}Au) in the 1950s.
  [Flocks R, *J Urol* **71**: 628–633, 1959]

- With the availability of gold-198 and iodine-125, several institutions reported on their experience using a retropubic 'free handed' approach, usually after patients underwent a lymph node dissection.
  [Zelefsy MJ, *J Urol* **158**: 23–30, 1997]
  [Schellhamer PF, *Urology* **56**: 436–441, 2000]

- This free-hand technique resulted in suboptimal distribution of seeds and poor dosimetry.
  [D'Amico A, *J Clin Oncol* **14**: 304–315, 1996]

- Researchers from Seattle initially described a closed transperineal implantation technique with the aid of transrectal ultrasonography (TRUS).
  - With this approach, the needles used to insert the radioactive seeds could be visualized, improving the accuracy of seed placement, compared with the retropubic approach, with a concomitant reduction in surgical morbidity and cost.
  [Holm H, *J Urol* **130**: 283–286, 1983]

- There are a number of different planning methods employed for permanent radioactive seed implantation.
  - The method popularized in Seattle calculates a dosimetric plan using pre-implantation TRUS images. These images are then used in the operating room to determine locations for planned seed placement.
  [Blasko J, *Semin Radiat Oncol* **3**: 240–249, 1993]

- A method was determined in which the dosimetric plan is calculated intraoperatively.
  [Kaplan I, *Int J Radiat Oncol Biol Phys* **42**(Suppl 1): 294, 1998]

- Others determined the number of seeds to be implanted based on the size of the gland and the nomogram (initially reported by Anderson).
  [Stone NJ, *Urology* **162**: 421–426, 1999]

- Other methods for seed implantation use computerized tomography (CT) guidance and an intraoperative magnetic resonance imaging (MRI) device.
  [Koutrouvelis P, *J Urol* **159**: 142–145, 1998]
  [D'Amico A, *Int J Radiat Oncol Biol Phys* **42**: 507–516, 1998]

- Postimplantation, CT can be performed both to determine seed localization and to reference the dose to the prostate and other structures of importance.
  [Willins J, *Int J Radiat Oncol Biol Phys* **39**: 347–353, 1997]

Isotopes

- There are several choices for isotopes for permanent seed implantation.

- Iodine-125 (^{125}I) is the most commonly used isotope.
  - It emits low-energy x-rays at 27 keV with a half-life of 59.6 days.

- Palladium-103 (^{103}Pd) was introduced in 1986.
  - The radiation emitted by palladium has an energy spectrum similar to that of iodine-125, with 21 keV x-rays, but it has a significantly shorter half-life of 17 days.

- Higher activity seeds are required for palladium-103 versus iodine-125 in order to deliver a similar tumoricidal dose (i.e. 1.3 μCi per palladium seed vs 0.4 μCi per iodine seed).

- There is also rapid fall-off at the borders of the implant when palladium-103 seeds are used.
  - This significantly ↓ the dose to normal structures such as the rectum and bladder.

- There are no published randomized trials that compare outcomes and toxicities of iodine-125 vs palladium-103.
  - There has been a tendency to implant patients with higher Gleason grades (specifically, Gleason grades > 8) with palladium, making retrospective analysis difficult.
  - In several series that controlled for presenting clinical prognostic variables, no difference in outcome was observed.
  - Some reports suggest that there are more acute urinary side-effects and less long-term toxicity with palladium-103.

Low dose rate brachytherapy as monotherapy

Outcomes

- Memorial Sloan Kettering Cancer Center Experience.
  [Zelefsky MJ, *Int J Radiat Oncol Biol Phys* **47**(5): 1261–1266, 2000]
  - Phase I/II prospective study accruing patients between 1988 and 1997.
  - 248 patients with T_{1c}–T_{2b} prostate cancer, with no evidence of nodal or distant metastasis, no previous pelvic radiation, and no previous transurethral resection of the prostate (TURP).
  - T_{1c} (143), T_{2a} (102), T_{2b} (3).
  - Median prostate-specific antigen (PSA) 7 ng/ml (range 1–58 ng/ml).
  - Gleason score < 6 (30), 6 (158), ≥ 7 (60).
  - A pre-implant CT scan was obtained, and computer-optimized dosimetry was undertaken for needle and source number and placement.
  - Median dose: 150 Gy (range 140–160 Gy).
  - Median activity: 45 mCi of iodine-125.
  - Median follow-up → 48 months (range 12–126 months).

- RESULTS:
  - 5-year relapse-free survival (RFS) for PSA: 0–4 ng/ml → 96%, 4–10 ng/ml → 84%, > 10 ng/ml → 62%.
  - Stratified into favorable (3 of 3), intermediate (2 of 3), and unfavorable risk (0 or 1 of 3) by PSA < 10 ng/ml, stage ≤ T_{2a}, and Gleason score ≤ 6.
  - Favorable risk 5-year RFS → 88%; intermediate risk 5-year RFS → 77%; unfavorable risk 5-year RFS 38%.
- SIDE-EFFECTS:
  - Acute urinary toxicity (Radiation Therapy Oncology Group (RTOG)) → grade 1 (40%); grade 2 (55%); grade 3 (3%).
  - Late urinary toxicity → grade 2 (40%); grade 3 (9%).
  - Rectal toxicity → grade 1 (33%); grade 2 (6%).
  - Impotency → 29%.
- CONCLUSIONS:
  - Excellent control of favorable risk.
  - PSA level and Gleason score are important variables.
  - Acceptable toxicity.
  - Urethral dose of 120–150% to keep toxicity low.
  - Higher impotency rates.

- Seattle Prostate Institute Experience with palladium-103. [Blasko JC, *Int J Radiat Oncol Biol Phys* **46**(4): 839–850, 2000]
  - Phase I/II prospective trial from January 1988 to December 1995.
  - 230 patients with moderately to poorly differentiated histology prostate cancer.
  - Median age: 69 years.
  - Median PSA: 7.3 ng/ml.
  - Gleason score ≥ 7 in 40%.
  - The prostate was defined using ultrasound scanning with a 2–5 mm margin, and preplanning and dosimetry.
  - 115 Gy was prescribed to the prostate volume with palladium-103 seeds.
  - Urethral dose was < 150%.
  - Median follow-up → 41.5 months.
  - RESULTS:
    - No evidence of disease (NED) → 90.9%; local failure → 3%; distant failure → 6.1%.
    - 5-year biochemical NED: Gleason 3–5 → (89%); Gleason 6 → (92%); Gleason 7 → (75%); Gleason 8–10 → (86%).
    - Stratified by Gleason 3–6 and PSA < 10 ng/ml.
    - Both are low risk, one is intermediate risk, and neither is high risk.

- 5-year biochemical NED: low risk, 94%; intermediate risk, 82%; high risk, 65%.
- SIDE-EFFECTS:
  - Toxicity not reported.
- CONCLUSIONS:
  - The palladium-103 transperineal implant gives excellent biochemical control of early stage, organ-confined prostate cancer.
  - The palladium-103 monotherapy implant provides excellent biochemical control in Gleason score 7, low PSA disease.

- Seattle Prostate Institute Experience with iodine-125.
  [Grimm PD, *Int J Radiat Oncol Biol Phys* **51**(1): 31–40, 2001]
  - Phase I/II prospective trial from January 1988 to December 1990.
  - 125 patients with low to moderate grade, early stage prostate cancer.
  - Treated with iodine-125 monotherapy implant.
  - Median age: 70 years.
  - The prostate was defined using ultrasound scanning, with preplanning and dosimetry.
  - Dose of 160 Gy (145 Gy TG-43, as per the American Association of Physicists in Medicine (AAPM) Task Force 43) prescribed to treatment volume.
  - Mean follow-up → 94.5 months.
  - RESULTS:
    - Overall PSA progression-free survival at 10 years → 87% for low-risk patients (PSA < 10 ng/ml, Gleason score 2–6, T_1–T_{2b}).
    - The 8 clinical failures occurred in the first 5 years.
    - The 8 biochemical failures occurred at a median of 52 months.
  - CONCLUSIONS:
    - Excellent control (87%) of low-risk prostate cancer with iodine-125 monotherapy implant at 10 years.
    - PSA decline is protracted over the life of the implant.
    - PSA and progression-free survival curves merge at 10 years.

Low dose rate brachytherapy in combination with external beam radiation therapy

- Seattle Prostate Institute Retrospective Review up until 1993.
  [Sylvester JE, *Int J Radiat Oncol Biol Phys* **57**(4): 944–952, 2003]
  - Retrospective review of patients receiving low dose rate (LDR) brachytherapy boost after external beam radiation therapy (EBRT) for prostate cancer from January 1987 to December 1993.

- 227 patients with neoadjuvant EBRT with iodine-125 or palladium-103 brachytherapy boost.
- Iodine-125 boost delivered at 120 Gy (108 TG-43).
- Palladium-103 boost delivered at 90 Gy (100 Gy NIST 1999, as per National Institutes of Standards and Technology (NIST)).
- Prostate volume was defined by ultrasound scanning with a 2–5 mm margin, with preplanning and dosimetry.
- Urethra was kept < 150%.
- EBRT was 45 Gy in 1.8-Gy fractions, with the four-field technique.
- Patients were stratified by PSA < 10 ng/ml, Gleason score 2–6, stage T_{1a}–T_{2b}.
- Patients were low risk if they met all three criteria, intermediate risk if they met two, and high risk if they met zero or one.
- Patients were low risk (27%), intermediate risk (40%), and high risk (33%).
- Mean follow-up → 63 months (range 4–172 months).
- RESULTS:
  - 13 patients had clinical failure (6%).
  - 10 patients had biochemical failure (4%).
  - 23 patients had distant failure (10%).
  - 165 patients were alive NED (73%).
  - Biochemical RFS of low-, intermediate-, and high-risk groups was 85%, 77%, and 45%, respectively.
- CONCLUSIONS:
  - Iodine-125 or palladium-103 brachytherapy for a boost after EBRT results in high rates of biochemical control.
  - High-risk patients need improvement of biochemical control.

High dose rate brachytherapy

[Vicini F, World J Urol 21(4): 220–228, 2003]
[Rodriguez RR, Hematol Oncol Clin North Am 13(3): 503–523, 1999]

Introduction

[Morton GC, Clin Oncol 17: 219–227, 2005]

- Several studies have demonstrated that radiation-dose escalation improves outcomes in patients with prostate cancer.
  [Zelefsky MJ, J Urol 166: 876–881, 2004]
  [Pollack A, Int J Radiat Oncol Biol Phys 53: 1097–1105, 2002]

- Delivery of high radiation doses requires techniques that spare normal tissue in order to avoid toxicity.

- Interstitial brachytherapy involves the insertion of radioactive sources into the prostate itself.
  - Because of a rapid dose fall-off beyond the prostate, normal tissue is spared.
  - However, disease beyond the capsule of the gland is potentially treated inconsistently.
  - For this reason, brachytherapy as a monotherapy should be primarily reserved for low-risk patients (PSA < 10 ng/ml, Gleason score ≤ 6, and stage I or II).

- Prostate brachytherapy can be performed with permanent LDR seeds (iodine-125 or palladium-103) or with high dose rate (HDR) temporary catheters (iridium-192).

- HDR brachytherapy usually involves the delivery of two or three large radiation fractions over a short period of time.
  - This differs from LDR permanent seed implants, which deliver their radiation over the course of months.

- From a radiobiological standpoint, treating prostate cancer with larger fraction sizes, such as those used in HDR treatment, offers a theoretical therapeutic advantage over LDR treatments.
  [Wang JZ, *Int J Radiat Oncol Biol Phys* **57**: 1101–1108, 2003]
  [Brenner DJ, *Int J Radiat Oncol Biol Phys* **52**: 6–13, 2002]
  [Fowler JF, *Int J Radiat Oncol Biol Phys* **56**: 1093–1103, 2003]

- The large radiation fractions used with HDR implants can potentially cause more damage to normal tissues.
  - However, HDR implants significantly improve the radiation dose distribution because of better control over the position of the source and the ability to vary the source dwell time, which is performed via intraoperative optimization.
  - This allows for better sparing of normal tissues, and resultant HDR implant toxicities have been found to be equivalent to LDR implant toxicities.

- HDR treatment for prostate cancer is still in its infancy, and there are currently few long-term outcome data.
  - Whether used in combination with EBRT or used as a monotherapy, total dose and fraction schemes vary greatly, making interstudy comparisons difficult.

High dose rate brachytherapy in combination with external beam radiation therapy

Introduction

- Most published reports using HDR brachytherapy involve EBRT with a brachytherapy boost.

- The EBRT is usually 45 Gy at 1.8 Gy per fraction.
  - The fractionation schedules published for the HDR vary, ranging from 1–2 fractions of 4–15 Gy per fraction.
  - In addition, the HDR component delivery sequence varies between studies; it has been given before, during, or after the EBRT, depending on the institution.

- The two most common fractionation approaches are:
  - Separate catheter insertions for each HDR fraction.
  - Single catheter insertion with the patient hospitalized, and 2–4 fractions given over 1–2 days.

- The multiple insertion technique requires multiple procedures; however, the single insertion, besides requiring a hospital stay, can lead to catheter migration.
  - Because of this migration, patient planning should be done separately for each fraction.
    [Damore SJ, Int J Radiat Oncol Biol Phys 46: 1205–1211, 2000]
    [Mullokandov E, Int J Radiat Oncol Biol Phys 58: 1063–1071, 2004]

- There are over 10 reported studies (almost all single institution) using combined EBRT and HDR brachytherapy.
    However, because of variations in patient selection, technique, fractionation, and biologically equivalent dose, interstudy comparison is difficult.
  - Presented below are those studies that have a median follow-up of > 30 months, in which the authors reported local control and disease-free survival (DFS) rates.

- RTOG 0321.
  - A phase II trial currently is investigating the use of 45 Gy EBRT with an HDR boost of 19 Gy in two fractions.
  - The RTOG study and a multicenter Canadian study are currently enrolling intermediate- and high-risk patients.
  - The goal is to establish further the safety and efficacy of this treatment, leading to a phase III study.

Outcomes

- Sahlgrenska University Hospital, Göteborg Series.
  [Borghede G, *Radiother Oncol* **44**: 237–244, 1997]
  - Study that accrued between July 1988 and June 1994.
  - Mean age: 63 years.
  - Included 50 patients, with T_{1b}–T_{3b} disease without distant metastasis, a prostate volume $< 60 \, cm^3$, and a life expectancy > 10 years, who underwent a staging lymphadenectomy.
  - T_1 (3), T_2 (34), T_3 (13) (lymph node (–) in 49/50 patients).
  - Pretreatment PSA level 0–4 (5), > 4–10 (25), > 10–20 (12), > 20 ng/ml (8).
  - Endocrine therapy not used until time of relapse, except in 1 patient.
  - Treatment was combination three-dimensional (3D) conformal EBRT (50 Gy) and HDR brachytherapy (2×10 Gy). EBRT was given for 2.5 weeks before and after HDR brachytherapy with the brachytherapy fractions given 2 weeks apart.
  - Local control measured by digital rectal examination (DRE), TRUS biopsy, and PSA evaluation.
  - Median follow-up → 45 months.
  - RESULTS:
    - Clinical biopsies verified local control in 48/50 (96%) patients; for stage T_1–T_2, 37/38 (97%); for stage T_3, 11/12 (92%).
    - At 45 months PSA < 1 ng/ml (39), PSA > 1–2 ng/ml (7), PSA > 4 ng/ml (4).
    - 48/50 patients were alive with/without recurrent or metastatic prostate cancer.
    - No patients died of prostate cancer, and both patients who did die had their prostate cancer locally controlled.
  - CONCLUSION:
    - Local control rates and minimal toxicity were promising, but longer follow-up is required.

- Long Beach Memorial Medical Center Series.
  [Syed AM, *Cancer Control* **8**: 511–521, 2001]
  - Study accrued between June 1996 and July 1999.
  - Mean age: 64 years.
  - 200 patients with T_{1c}–T_{3b} disease, without distant metastasis, with a prostate volume of $< 60 \, cm^3$, and a life expectancy of > 10 years, who underwent a staging lymphadenectomy.
  - T_1, 28 patients; T_2, 129 patients; T_3, 43 patients.
  - Gleason score 0–4, 28 patients; 5–7, 151 patients; 8–10, 21 patients.

- Pretreatment average PSA: 10 ng/ml.
- Endocrine therapy, involving monthly leuprolide, was given to patients with a Gleason score 8–10 or PSA > 20 ng/ml (72 patients).
- Treatment given by combination 3D conformal EBRT (39.6 Gy for T_{1c}/T_{2a}; 45 Gy for T_{2b}/T_3) and HDR brachytherapy (22–26 Gy in 4 fractions).
- EBRT was initiated 2–3 weeks after HDR brachytherapy, with brachytherapy given in 4 fractions over 2 days.
- Local control was defined as complete resolution of nodule, or induration following completion of irradiation.
- Median follow-up → 30 months.
- RESULTS:
  - Clinically verified local control in 194/200 (97%) patients.
  - Cause-specific survival rate → 97%.
  - At 25 months PSA < 1 ng/ml (170 patients), > 1–2 ng/ml (22 patients), > 2 ng/ml (8 patients).
- SIDE-EFFECTS:
  - No late grade 4/5 toxicities.
  - Late grade 3 genitourinary toxicity → 2%; grade 3 gastrointestinal toxicities → 1.5%.
- CONCLUSIONS:
  - HDR brachytherapy with EBRT is well tolerated, with a PSA relapse-free survival of 97%, which is favorable compared with other modalities.
  - The local control rate is subjective, as it was based solely on DRE.

- Berlin Multi-institutional Study Series.
  [Deger S, *Eur Urol* **41**: 420–426, 2002]
  - Study that accrued between December 1992 and December 1997.
  - Mean age: 67.3 years.
  - 230 patients with T_1–T_3 disease, without lymph node or distant metastasis, who underwent staging lymphadenectomy.
  - T_1, 16 patients; T_2, 80 patients; T_3, 134 patients.
  - Median pretreatment PSA: 12.8 ng/ml.
  - Treatment given by combination EBRT (40 Gy) and HDR brachytherapy (2 × 10 Gy given 1 week apart). After December 1993, the HDR dose was changed to 9 Gy/fraction and the EBRT dose to 45 (T_1/T_2) and 50.4 Gy (T_3).
  - Local control measured by DRE, TRUS biopsy, and PSA evaluation.
  - Median follow-up → 40 months.

- RESULTS:
  - 5-year overall survival → 93%.
  - 5-year cause-specific survival → 98%.
  - Median PSA at 5 years: 0.18 ng/ml.
  - No residual disease seen in 50% of biopsies at 1 year ($n = 128$) and 68% of biopsies at 2 years ($n = 77$).
  - Disease failures consisted of 21 local only, 12 systemic only, and 8 local + systemic.
- SIDE-EFFECTS:
  - Late grade 3 or 4 complications occurred in 12% of patients.
  - All patients had undergone TURP or urethrotomy in the previous year.
- CONCLUSIONS:
  - ↓ HDR fraction dose from 10 to 9 Gy may have led to less toxicity.
  - No grade 3 or 4 toxicities developed after changing the fractionation scheme.
  - Complication rates were comparable to LDR brachytherapy.
  - Local control data are difficult to compare with other studies because not all patients underwent repeat biopsy.

- William Beaumont Hospital Series.
  [Martinez AA, *Int J Radiat Oncol Biol Phys* **53**: 316–327, 2002]
  - Dose escalation study that accrued between November 1991 and August 2000.
  - Median age: 68 years.
  - 311 (104 ineligible, giving a total 207) patients, with expected survival > 5 years, prostate volume ≤ 65 cm^3, age < 85 years, PSA ≥ 10 ng/ml, Gleason score ≥ 7, or clinical stage $\geq T_{2b}$.
  - No patients received androgen suppression.
  - Patients underwent repeat TRUS biopsy if they had not developed metastatic disease.
  - T_{1c}–T_{2a}, 30%; T_{2b}, 28%; T_{2c}, 32%; T_3, 10%.
  - Mean pretreatment PSA: 11.5 ng/ml.
  - Treatment given by combination EBRT (46 Gy) and interdigitated HDR brachytherapy.
    - Initial HDR fraction was 5.5 Gy, then 6 Gy, then 6.5 Gy in 3 fractions (low dose group, 28%).
    - After October 1995, 2 fractions were given at 8.25, 8.75, 9.5, 10.5, and then 11.5 Gy, in succession (high dose group, 72%).
    - Total biologically equivalent dose: 80.2–136.3 Gy.
  - Local control measured by DRE, TRUS biopsy, and PSA evaluation.

- Median follow-up → 4.4 years.
- RESULTS:
  - 5-year overall survival: low dose, 93%; high dose, 91%; $p = 0.745$.
  - 5-year cause-specific survival: low dose, 95%; high dose, 100%; $p = 0.014$.
  - 5-year DFS: low dose, 50%; high dose, 77%; $p < 0.001$.
  - Median PSA at 5 years → 0.18 ng/ml.
- SIDE-EFFECTS:
  - 5-year late grade 3 and 4 gastrointestinal and genitourinary complications occurred in 0.5% and 0.5%, and 8% and 0%, respectively.
- CONCLUSIONS:
  - EBRT interdigitated with HDR brachytherapy boost proved an effective treatment for unfavorable prostate cancers.
  - A therapeutic advantage was demonstrated with higher brachytherapy doses.
  - Complication rates were favorable.

- Christian-Albrechts University, Kiel Services.
  [Kovács G, *Cancer Radiother* 7: 100–106, 2003]
  - Study that accrued between February 1986 and September 1996.
  - Median age → 68 years.
  - 144 patients with prostate volume < 70 cm^3, N_0M_0 by bone scan and CT or MRI.
  - T_{1b}–T_{2a}, 20.1% patients; T_{2c}–T_3, 79.9% patients.
  - 54 (37.5%) patients received < 6 months of hormonal ablation.
  - Mean pretreatment PSA: 11.5 ng/ml.
  - Treatment given by combination EBRT (50 Gy) and 2 fractions of interdigitated HDR brachytherapy (9–10 Gy ×2 fractions; 2–3 week interval between fractions).
  - Median follow-up → 8 years.
  - RESULTS:
    - Overall survival → 71.5%.
    - No biochemical evidence of disease → 72.9%.
    - DFS → 82.6%.
  - SIDE-EFFECTS:
    - Late grade 3 genitourinary and gastrointestinal toxicities occurred in 2.3% and 4.1%, respectively.
    - No late grade 4 toxicities were documented.
  - CONCLUSIONS:
    - EBRT with HDR brachytherapy was an effective treatment for localized prostate cancer, especially high-risk cases.

- The influence of androgen ablation on outcome was not determinable.

Summary of studies: HDR brachytherapy + EBRT

Author	Center/ series	No. of patients	Median follow-up (months)	Local control (%)	Disease-free survival (%)
Borghede	Göteborg	50	45	96	84
Syed	Long Beach	200	30	97	93
Deger	Berlin	230	40	99	98
Martinez	William Beaumont	207	53	98	68
Kovács	Kiel	144	96	91	82.6

Outcomes involving androgen deprivation

- There are limited prospective data comparing HDR boost with EBRT with or without androgen deprivation.

- Listed below are the outcomes of two separate studies; however, these studies used, in part, a pooled patient population.

- [Martinez AA, J Urol **170**: 2296–2301, 2003]
  - 507 patients accrued between 1986 and 2000 at two centers.
    - Kiel (198 patients) and William Beaumont (309 patients).
  - Patient eligibility was a pretreatment PSA > 10 ng/ml and Gleason score > 7.
  - > cT_{2b}, and maximum prostate volume 65 cm³.
  - Patients were treated with HDR brachytherapy interdigitated with EBRT (46 Gy).
  - HDR dose was increased from 5.5 Gy ×3 fractions to 15 Gy ×2 fractions.
  - 177 patients received androgen-suppression therapy (AST); the remaining 330 patients did not receive AST.
  - AST was given over 6 months, neoadjuvantly and concurrently.
  - Mean patient age → 68 years.
  - Mean follow-up → 4.8 years.

- RESULTS:

	8-year overall survival	8-year cause- specific survival	8-year disease- free survival	8-year biochemical control	8-year local recurrence
No AST	76%	94%*	59%	75%	10.8
AST	75%	86%	60%	66%	9.2

*Statistically significant.

- CONCLUSIONS:
  - The trial showed high overall and cause-specific survival as well as low biochemical failures.
  - For intermediate- and high-risks patients there was no added benefit from short course (6 months) AST.
  - The authors concluded that with high biologically equivalent doses there may be no need for adjuvant AST.
  - The benefit of AST in this group of patients, which was seen in previous phase III EBRT studies, may have been related to the older techniques and relatively low doses of EBRT used.

- [Martinez AA, *Int J Radiat Oncol Biol Phys* **62**:1322–1331, 2005]
  - 934 patients accrued between 1986 and 2000 at three centers.
    - Kiel (198 patients), William Beaumont (315 patients), and California Endocurietherapy (459 patients).
  - Patient eligibility was a pretreatment PSA > 10 ng/ml, Gleason score > 7, > cT_{2b}, and maximum prostate volume 65 cm^3.
  - Patients were treated with HDR brachytherapy interdigitated with EBRT (36–50 Gy).
  - HDR dose was escalated from 5.5 Gy ×3 fractions to 15 Gy ×2 fractions.
  - 406 patients received AST, with the remaining 528 patients not receiving AST.
  - AST was given over 6 months, neoadjuvantly and concurrently.
  - Mean patient age → 69 years.
  - Mean follow-up → 4.4 years.
  - RESULTS:

	8-year overall survival	8-year cause- specific survival	8-year biochemical control
No AST	78%	94%	81%
AST	83%	89%	85%

- CONCLUSIONS:
  - For intermediate- and high-risk patients there was no added benefit from short-course (6 months) AST, but there were added costs and side-effects.
  - The authors question the use of short term AST with high-dose radiation.

Summary of studies: androgen deprivation

Study	No. of patients	Follow-up (years)	8-year biochemical control (AST/no AST)	8-year disease-free survival (AST/no AST)
Martinez (2003)	507	4.8	66%/75%	60%/59%
Martinez (2005)	934	4.4	85%/81%	

High dose rate brachytherapy as monotherapy

Introduction

- HDR brachytherapy as a monotherapy is still in its infancy.

- The radiobiologic argument supporting HDR monotherapy use in prostate cancer is the same as for using an HDR boost in combination with EBRT.

- Because this form of therapy only treats the prostate gland itself, most proponents support its use in low-risk patients.

- Although this method is very promising, limited data available at this time. Three of the four published studies are summarized below.

Outcomes

- Osaka University Series.
  [Yoshioka Y, *Int J Radiat Oncol Biol Phys* 48: 675–681, 2000]
  - Phase I/II prospective study that accrued between January 1994 and September 1998.
  - 22 patients with T_1–T_4 (bladder neck invasion) without nodal or distant metastasis, with no previous pelvic radiation, prior surgery/ TURP to prostate gland, or prostate cancer recurrence.

- T_1, 4 patients; T_2, 6 patients; T_3, 9 patients; T_4, 3 patients.
- Median PSA → 30.9 ng/ml.
- Patients with a PSA > 20 ng/ml or T_3/T_4 disease received neoadjuvant hormone therapy (19 patients) with a leuteinizing hormone releasing hormone (LHRH) agonist and antiandrogen.
- No patients received any EBRT or surgery.
- Transperineal needle implants were performed using real-time ultrasound guidance with a perineal template, followed by CT simulation.
  - Median number of needles used was 16 (range 8–18).
- Treatment involved twice daily irradiation with a time interval of 6 hours.
- Total dose was 48 Gy in 8 fractions over 5 days (first 7 cases) or 54 Gy in 9 fractions over 5 days (last 15 cases).
- The dose to the urethra ranged between 54 and 81 Gy, and the dose to the anterior mucosa surface of the rectum was < 54 Gy.
- Median follow-up → 31 months.
- RESULTS:
  - There were no significant intra- or perioperative complications.
  - There were no grade 3 or higher toxicities.
  - PSA levels normalized within 20 months of irradiation in 95% of patients.
  - 4-year clinical and biochemical relapse-free rates → 95% and 55%, respectively.
- CONCLUSION:
  - This early study demonstrated acceptable toxicity, with short-term outcomes comparable to those with LDR treatments.

- [Martinez AA, *Int J Radiat Oncol Biol Phys* **49**: 61–69, 2001]
  - Phase II, prospective study that accrued between March 1999 and June 2000 (William Beaumont Hospital).
  - 41 patients with low- and selected intermediate-risk prostate cancer (Gleason score < 7, PSA < 10 ng/ml, stage < T_{2a}).
  - Median pretreatment PSA 4.7 ng/ml; Gleason score (GS) 5, 3 patients; GS 6, 33 patients; GS 7, 4 patients.
  - No patients underwent any EBRT or surgery.
  - Median age → 64 years.
  - Transperineal needle implants were placed using a template with TRUS guidance.
    - An interactive, real-time planning system with geometric optimization was used.
  - Total dose 38 Gy in 4 fractions delivered twice daily over 2 days.

- The dose to any segment of the urethra or rectum was restrained to $< 75\%$ and $< 125\%$ of the prescription dose, respectively.
- Median follow-up not reported; minimum follow-up $\rightarrow$ 4 months.
- RESULTS:
  - No significant intra- or perioperative complications.
  - No grade 3 or higher toxicities; 5 patients had grade 2 toxicity (3 genitourinary and 2 gastrointestinal).
  - No late toxicities or control rates reported.
- CONCLUSION:
  - Study supports the feasibility of and acceptable acute toxicities of HDR monotherapy.

- [Grills IA, *J Urol* **171**: 1098–1104, 2004]
  - Phase II/III, non-randomized, prospective study accrued over 1999–2001 (William Beaumont Hospital).
  - 149 patients with low-risk prostate cancer (Gleason score < 6, PSA < 10 ng/ml, stage $< T_{2a}$).
  - Gleason score (GS): GS < 5, 9 patients; GS 6, 135 patients; GS 7, 5 patients.
  - No patients underwent EBRT or surgery.
  - 36% of patients underwent neoadjuvant hormone manipulation for gland-size optimization.
  - Stratification:
    - Group I ($n = 65$): HDR brachytherapy, 38 Gy in 4 fractions delivered twice daily over 2 days.
    - Group II ($n = 84$): LDR brachytherapy (^{103}Pd), 120 Gy.
  - Median age $\rightarrow$ 70 years.
  - Median follow-up $\rightarrow$ 35 months.
  - RESULTS:
    - Biochemical control was 97% and 98% for LDR and HDR brachytherapy, respectively.
    - HDR brachytherapy was associated with significant $\downarrow$ in rates of acute dysuria, urinary frequency, and rectal pain, as well as chronic frequency and urgency and impotence.
  - CONCLUSIONS:
    - HDR brachytherapy maintained the same biochemical control as LDR in a short follow-up (3 years).
    - HDR monotherapy gave a significant $\downarrow$ in rates of acute and chronic toxicities compared with LDR.

15

Radical prostatectomy

- The widespread use of prostate-specific antigen (PSA) testing, along with the generalized ↑ in the public awareness of prostate cancer, have allowed for progressively earlier detection of ♂ with prostate cancer over the last 25 years.

- Recent work from the Cancer of the Prostate Strategic Urologic Research Endeavor (CaPSURE) has documented this stage migration, in which the number of ♂ presenting with low- and intermediate-risk prostate cancer has ↑ from 62% → 84% over the period 1989–2002. [Cooperberg MR, *J Clin Oncol* **23**: 8146–8151, 2005]

- These low- and intermediate-risk groups of patients with prostate cancer may be the ones most likely to benefit from aggressive local therapy.
  - They are also the most likely groups to undergo radical prostatectomy.
    [Cooperbereg MR, *J Urol* **171**: 1398–1401, 2004]

Indications

- Treatment options for clinically localized prostate cancer include:
  - Radical prostatectomy.
  - Radiation therapy.
  - Active surveillance.

- The American Urological Association (AUA) prostate cancer guidelines panel established the following treatment recommendations in their 1995 report on prostate cancer:
  [Middleton RG, *J Urol* **154**: 2144–2148, 1995]

- An assessment of the patient's life expectancy, overall health status, and tumor characteristics is necessary before any treatment decisions for prostate cancer can be made.
- The patient should be informed about currently accepted initial interventions, which include radical prostatectomy, radiation therapy, and surveillance.
- Patient preference for a particular treatment option, which is based on his attitude toward the course of the disease and the benefits and harms of the different interventions, should be considered in determining his treatment.
- Data from the literature do not provide clear-cut evidence for the superiority of any one treatment.

- Recent data have emerged that demonstrate possible advantages of radical prostatectomy over surveillance in selected patients with newly diagnosed prostate cancer:

- The Scandinavian Prostatic Cancer Study Group.
  [Holmberg L, *N Engl J Med* **347**(11): 781–789, 2002]
  [Bill-Axelson A, *N Engl J Med* **352**(19): 1977–1984, 2005]
  - Patients with localized prostate cancer were randomized to treatment with either radical prostatectomy ($n = 347$) or watchful waiting ($n = 348$).
  - Between 1988 and 1999.
  - Mean follow-up → 8.2 years.
  - RESULTS:
    - Patients undergoing radical prostatectomy have significant advantages in terms of cancer-specific survival, development of distant metastases, local progression, the need for initiation of hormone therapy, palliative radiation therapy, and the requirement for laminectomy.
  - CONCLUSIONS:
    - Despite these compelling data, there is still no difference in overall survival between the two study groups, and a total of 27% of patients have died.
    - This important study confirms the importance of competing causes of mortality, which must be weighed up when deciding on a treatment strategy for an individual patient.
  - LIMITATIONS OF THE STUDY:
    - Only 5% of the cancers in this study were detected by screening, > 75% were palpable, stage $\geq T_2$, and ~ 50% had PSA > 10.0 ng/ml.

- Therefore, these results may not be as profound when applied to the majority of contemporary patients, who are more likely to be clinical stage T_{1c} with a PSA < 10 ng/ml.
  [Cooperberg MR, *J Clin Oncol* **23**: 8146–8151, 2005]

History

- A review of all the technical modifications that have been made to optimize oncologic control and reduce the perioperative morbidity associated with radical prostatectomy is beyond the scope of this text.

- However, the description of the anatomy of Santorini's plexus and the branches of the pelvic plexus that innervate the corpora cavernosa were critical to the development of an organized and anatomically based surgical approach to radical retropubic prostatectomy.
  [Reiner WG, *J Urol* **121**: 198–200, 1979]
  [Walsh PC, *J Urol* **128**: 492–497, 1982]

- This approach emphasizes:
  - The surgical management of the dorsal vein complex.
  - The meticulous dissection of the prostatic apex.
  - Preservation of the neurovascular bundles.
  - A precise urethrovesical anastomosis.

- An understanding of the anatomic landmarks that have been defined over the last 20 years are essential in performing a successful radical prostatectomy. These landmarks are displayed in Fig. 15.1.

- Numerous modifications to the technique have been incorporated into our adaptation of this procedure; the University of Miami technique is described below.

The University of Miami radical prostatectomy

Anesthesia

- Regional anesthesia (spinal or epidural) has been associated with less blood loss and a lower frequency of pulmonary emboli in patients undergoing radical prostatectomy.
  [Peters C, *J Urol* **134**: 81–83, 1985]
  [Shir Y, *Urology* **45**: 993, 1995]

- A single administration of intrathecal opioids has several advantages over epidural analgesia, including faster onset of action, technical

155

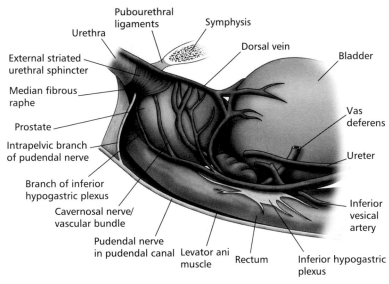

Fig. 15.1 Anatomical landmarks of the prostate necessary in understanding radical prostatectomy.

ease of administration, lower cost, and little delay in postoperative ambulation.
[Eandi JA, *Prostate Cancer Prostatic Dis* **5**: 226–230, 2002]
[Gottschalk A, *JAMA* **279**: 1076–1082, 1998]
[Stoelting RK, *Anesth Analg* **68**: 707–709, 1989]
[Gardner TA, *Cancer* **89**: 424–430, 2000]

- In addition to improvement in perioperative pain scores and diminished intraoperative blood loss, a recent randomized, controlled trial demonstrated that spinal anesthesia was also associated with earlier passage of flatus and a faster postoperative recovery time than general anesthesia.
[Salonia A, *Urology* **64**(1): 95–100, 2004]

Incision

- The patient is placed in the supine position on the operating table.
  - The kidney rest is elevated under the ischial tuberosities, and the table is flexed in order to extend the distance between the pubis and the umbilicus.
  - Sequential pneumatic compression stockings are placed prior to the incision.

- Once the patient has been prepared and draped, a 16-French, Foley catheter is placed and filled with 30 ml of sterile water. Traditionally, a midline lower abdominal, extraperitoneal incision is used.
  - In recent years we have routinely used a modified transverse Pfannenstiel incision.
    [Manoharan M, *Urology* **64**(2): 369–371, 2004]
- Once the rectus fascia has been incised, the rectus muscles are separated at the midline, and the transversalis fascia is opened. This provides a direct route to the space of Retzius.
  - The fibrofatty tissue overlying the pelvic side walls is gently dissected using sharp and blunt dissection. This allows for visualization of the external iliac vein and spermatic cord laterally. It also allows for cephalad mobilization of the peritoneum.
  - Mobilization of the peritoneum may be more challenging in patients who have undergone prior hernia repair.
  - An inadvertent peritoneotomy can be closed with a running chromic catgut suture.

Lymphadenectomy

- A Buchwalter retractor is placed, and a bilateral pelvic lymph node dissection may be performed at this time.
  - Traditionally, pelvic lymphadenectomy has implied the removal of all node-bearing tissue from the circumflex iliac vessels distally, to the bifurcation of the common iliac vessels proximally.
  - The lymphadenectomy extends superiorly to the external iliac vein, and laterally to the pelvic side wall.
  - The lymphadenectomy extends inferiorly to the obturator nerve, which is dissected free from the surrounding lymph-node-containing tissue.
  - Hemoclips or sutures are placed on larger lymphatic trunks in order to prevent subsequent lymphocele formation.
  - Great care is exercised when dissecting around the obturator nerve, which permits adduction of the lower extremities at the hip.
- There has clearly been an evolution in the rationale for pelvic lymphadenectomy, which is largely reflected in the anatomical boundaries that it encompasses.
  - Once thought to be curative, particularly in patients with low-volume metastatic disease, the boundaries of the extended lymphadenectomy included node-bearing tissue in the areas surrounding

the external iliac artery, the genitofemoral nerve, and even within the presacral space.
[Golimbu M, *J Urol* **121**: 617–620, 1979]

- Due to the stage migration that has occurred as a result of the widespread use of PSA testing, as well as a better selection of surgical candidates for surgery, there has been a decline in the number of patients who are found to have nodal metastases at the time of radical prostatectomy.
  [Petros JA, *J Urol* **147**: 1574–1575, 1992]
  - As a result, a modified, more limited lymphadenectomy has been adopted by most surgeons.
  - This serves primarily as a staging procedure, because resection of positive lymph nodes rarely results in any long-term oncologic control.
- However, some studies cite advantages of a more extensive lymphadenectomy, including:
  - Removal of more lymph nodes.
  - Detection of more lymph node metastases.
  - A higher PSA-free progression rate in patients with limited lymph node metastases.
    [Allaf ME, *J Urol* **172**(5 Pt 1): 1840–1844, 2004]
- Other studies, however, have suggested that the extent of the lymph node dissection does not affect PSA progression, and can be omitted in patients with PSA < 10 ng/ml, a Gleason score ≤ 6, and stage T_{1c} or T_{2a} disease.
  [DiMarco DS, *J Urol* **173**: 1121–1125, 2005]
  [Bhatta-Dhar N, *Urology* **63**(3): 528–531, 2004]

Dorsal vein and apical dissection

- The endopelvic fascia is opened sharply and bilaterally from the apex to the base of the prostate.
  - The puboprostatic ligaments, which can be seen at the superior edges of the endopelvic fascia, are treated with great care, and are usually not transected or torn.
  - Sparing of the periurethral striated muscle, as well as the supporting structures such as the puboprostatic ligaments, is important for the preservation of continence.
    [Poore RE, *Urology* **51**: 67–72, 1998]
    [Jarrow JP, *Semin Urol Oncol* **18**: 28–32, 2000]
    [Steiner MS, *Semin Urol Oncol* **18**: 9–18, 2000]
    [Eastham JA, *J Urol* **156**: 1707–1713, 1996]

- Once the endopelvic fascia has been opened, the levator muscle attachments to the prostate are gently teased off the prostate.
  - Small perforating vessels should be divided between hemoclips. The edges of the endopelvic fascia are grasped between allis clamps, and 'bunching sutures' are placed over the dorsal aspect of the prostate at the bladder neck.
  - These absorbable sutures limit back-bleeding from the bladder side of the dorsal vein complex, and allow for better exposure of the prostatic apex.

- After two sutures have been placed just above the apex of the prostate, electrocautery is used to divide the dorsal vein complex just cephalad to the apex of the prostate.
  - Using sustained downward pressure on the midportion of the prostate with a sponge stick, metzenbaum scissors are used to develop a plane between the anterior fibromuscular stroma and the deep dorsal vein complex (Fig. 15.2).

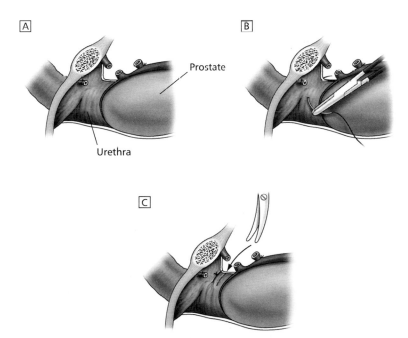

Fig. 15.2 Division of the deep dorsal vein complex. Following the contour of the anterior fibromuscular stroma allows for preservation of the puboprostate ligaments and striated sphincter complex.

- Hemoclips are used sparingly to control some of the small perforators on the lateral aspect of the dorsal vein complex, and great care is taken to maintain close proximity to the anterior fibromuscular stroma while dissecting distally toward the prostatourethral junction. Alternatively, a harmonic scalpel can be used to divide the tissue lateral to the urethra.
- We believe that remaining close to the fibromuscular stroma, which rarely contains tumor, avoids disturbing the pubourethral component of the puboprostatic ligaments. These bands may contribute significantly to postoperative continence.

• Once the apex of the prostate has been cleared medially and distally, dissection proceeds directly down onto the urethra.
- The apex of the prostate is carefully dissected sharply from the remaining levator muscle attachments.
- A transverse incision is made in the anterior portion of the urethra, exposing the Foley catheter (Fig. 15.3).
- The anterior row of sutures, corresponding to the 10, 12, and 2 o'clock positions, are then sequentially placed on the urethral stump (see Fig. 15.3).
- Once these sutures have been placed, the distal end of the Foley catheter is completely divided just beyond the urethral meatus. It is then fed up through the anterior urethral opening and grasped with a Kelly clamp in order to prevent loss of fluid from the balloon, which is situated in the urinary bladder.

• If a nerve-sparing procedure is planned, the periprostatic fascia along the lateral aspects of the prostate is incised.

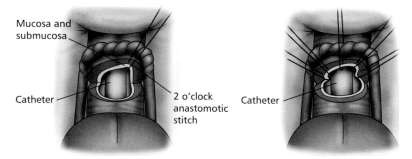

Fig. 15.3 The anterior urethra is incised and the first series of anterior urethral anastomotic sutures are placed.

- The neurovascular bundles are then sharply dissected off the lateral aspects of the prostate.
- Dissection of the neurovascular bundles is performed with metzenbaum scissors, and hemoclips are placed on small perforators that enter the prostate laterally.
- We avoid the use of electocautery, which may induce thermal injury to these structures.
- The neurovascular bundles are freed both proximally and distally along the lateral aspects of the prostatic apex.
- The use of optical loupes may facilitate this part of the procedure.

Dissection of the prostate off of the rectum

- The posterior urethra is then divided with full visualization of the mobilized neurovascular bundles.
  - A plane behind the posterior leaf of Denonvillier's fascia is developed at the midline by first taking down the posterior urethral plate and rectourethralis muscles sharply (Fig. 15.4).
  - The posterior lip of the prostate may extend in a caudal direction, and care should be taken to avoid entering the prostate gland posteriorly.
    [Myers RP, Urol Clin N Am **18**: 211–227, 1991]

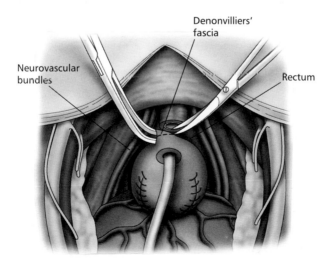

Denonvilliers' fascia

Neurovascular bundles

Rectum

Fig. 15.4 Following release of the neurovascular bundles, the posterior urethral plate, rectourethralis, and posterior leaf of Denonvillier's fascia are transected.

- The lateral pelvic fascia is sequentially divided in a cephalad direction, allowing the prostate to be delivered superiorly (Fig. 15.5).
- Great care must be exercised, particularly when the more cephalad portions of the lateral pelvic fascia are being separated from the prostate, in order to avoid inadvertent injury to the neurovascular bundles.

• Once the prostate has been fully lifted off the anterior rectal wall, Denonvillier's fascia is incised just above the base of the prostate and the bladder neck, allowing for dissection of the bilateral vasa deferens and seminal vesicles.

- The prostatic vascular pedicles are now divided just lateral to the seminal vesicles, using either suture or the harmonic scalpel, again taking great care to avoid injury to the neurovascular bundles.

The base and bladder neck

• The seminal vesicles are dissected distally to their apex, where a hemoclip is placed on the artery of the seminal vesicle.

- The vas are divided, with electrocautery.

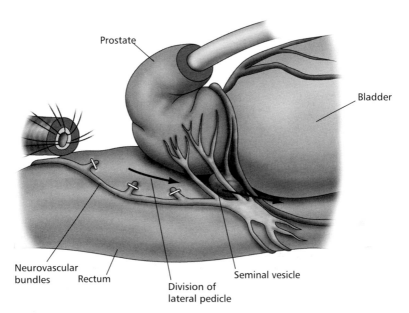

Fig. 15.5 The lateral pelvic fascia is gently released, with great care, to avoid injury to the neurovascular bundles.

- Dissection of the prostate from the bladder neck can be done using either a standard anterior wide excision or via bladder-neck-sparing techniques. These bladder-neck-preserving techniques provide for preservation of the circular fibers of the bladder neck, which may provide for improved early postoperative continence in ♂ undergoing radical prostatectomy.
  [Shelfo SW, *Urology* **51**: 73–78, 1998]
  [Soloway MS, *Semin Urol Oncol* **18**: 51–56, 2000]
  [Deliveliotis C, *Urology* **60**: 855–858, 2002]
- Bladder-neck preservation may ↑ the (+) margin rate of radical prostatectomy by 3–10%.
  [Brasilis KG, *Eur Urol* **28**: 202–208, 1995]
  [Srougi M, *J Urol* **165**: 815–818, 2001]
- However, we and others have found that the bladder neck is rarely a sole (+) margin in these cases.
  [Wieder J, *J Urol* **160**(2): 299–315, 1998]
  [Bianco FJ, *Eur Urol* **43**: 461–466, 2003]

- A tennis-racquet closure of the bladder neck may be performed at this time if bladder-neck preservation has not been performed.
  - Frozen sections of the apex or the bladder neck may be selectively taken at this time, if needed.
    [Shah O, *J Urol* **165**(6 Pt 1): 1943–1948, 2001]
  - This may provide additional information for determining whether wider excision of these structures needs to be performed, particularly in patients with more advanced tumors.

The anastomosis

- Once hemostasis has been achieved, the neurovascular bundles and the anterior rectal wall are assessed, and finally an anastomosis is performed between the urethra and the bladder neck (Fig. 15.6).
  - The remaining four posterior sutures in the urethra are placed at the 3 and 9 o'clock positions, and the 5 and 7 o'clock positions with double-armed needles.
  - Sutures are placed first in the urethra, using double-armed needles. The opposite ends of the sutures are then placed on the bladder neck in their respective positions.
  - A 20-French, Foley catheter is placed through the anastomosis, and the sutures are tied down, sealing the anastomosis around the catheter.
  - Irrigation of sterile saline through the Foley catheter may be done to test the integrity of the anastomosis.

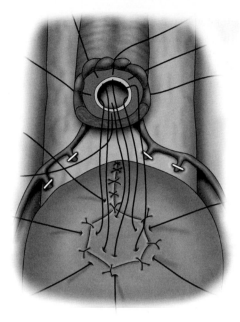

Fig. 15.6 The anastomosis is performed between the bladder neck and the urethra.

- A closed suction drain may be placed for a short period of time following surgery, although this may be omitted in patients with no evidence of urinary leak from the anastomosis.
  [Savoie M, *J Urol* **170**(1): 112–114, 2003]

Outcome measures for radical prostatectomy

Oncologic efficacy of radical prostatectomy

- The serum PSA should ↓ to undetectable levels within 2–3 weeks following a radical prostatectomy.
  - We have used a serum PSA level of < 0.2 ng/ml in order to confirm treatment success.
  - Supersensitive assays have become available and may allow for PSA detection at lower levels.
- Persistence of a detectable PSA following radical prostatectomy implies either:
  - The presence of retained benign prostatic tissue.
  - Persistence of residual local tumor.
  - The presence of metastatic disease.

- PSA failure following radical prostatectomy is a surrogate endpoint in patients with prostate cancer, and in many cases will antedate the development of metastatic disease, and subsequently death, from prostate cancer.
  [Pound CR, JAMA **17**: 1591–1597, 1999]
  - The evaluation and management of a rising PSA following radical prostatectomy is discussed in Chapters 16 and 19.

- Table 15.1 provides 5-, 10-, and 15-year follow-up data for three of the largest contemporary radical prostatectomy series. Particularly within the early years of each of these studies, a large number of patients with poor adverse prognostic indicators were treated surgically. Features such as PSA values > 10 ng/ml, bulky clinical stage (including T_3 tumors), and high Gleason scores have undoubtedly adversely impacted the overall PSA recurrence in these studies. Subgroup analyses of these studies have confirmed that patients with low and intermediate risk, based on their initial PSA level, Gleason score, and T stage, have considerably higher PSA-free survival.

- While these data are representative of radical prostatectomy outcomes in high volume, academic centers of excellence, recent studies have

Table 15.1 Long-term efficacy of radical prostatectomy: biochemical and cancer-specific survival in several large contemporary series

Series	No. of patients	5-, 10-, 15-year data	
		PSA-free progression (%)	Cancer-specific survival (%)
[Han M, *Urol Clin North Am* 28(3): 555–565, 2001]	2,404	84/74/66	99/96/90
[Zincke H, *J Urol* **152**(5 Pt 2): 1850–1857,1994]	3,170	70/52/40	NS/90/82
[Bianco FJ, *Urology* 66(Suppl 5A): 83–94, 2005]	1,746	82/77/75	99/95/89

NS, not specified.

questioned whether these data can be reproduced by those who perform fewer radical prostatectomies.

- A study evaluated a cohort of over 12,600 Medicare beneficiaries who underwent radical prostatectomy.
[Ellison LM, *J Urol* **173**: 2094–2098, 2005]
- RESULTS:
  - Low-volume radical prostatectomy centers (defined as performing < 33 procedures per year) selected patients more likely to be cured by radical prostatectomy, based on the preoperative PSA, T stage, and Gleason score.
  - Despite this, patients treated at low-volume centers had a 17% ↑ hazard ratio of receiving adjuvant therapy.
  - Difference in surgical technique is one explanation for these findings.

Prognostic variables associated with radical prostatectomy

- The most widely accepted pretreatment variables that predict the final pathologic stage at the time of the radical prostatectomy include: pretreatment PSA, clinical T stage, and the Gleason score of the prostate biopsy.

- These factors have been incorporated in a series of nomograms, which were later updated and validated using data obtained from 4,133 ♂ undergoing radical prostatectomy at one of three different institutions.
[Partin AW, *JAMA* **277**(18): 1445–1451, 1997]

- The distinction between tumors with a Gleason score of $3 + 4 = 7$ and those with a Gleason score of $4 + 3 = 7$, in terms of the impact that this has on final histology, has been recently addended to the updated nomograms.
[Partin AW, *Urology* **58**: 843–848, 2001]

- While the serum PSA, T stage, and Gleason score may predict the final pathologic stage of the tumor at the time of radical prostatectomy, additional variables have been found to be important in predicting the patient's overall prognosis following radical prostatectomy.
  - Using the margin status, final pathologic stage, and primary and secondary Gleason grades within the final prostate specimen, a continuous multivariable postoperative nomogram was developed and later updated, which predicts the 10-year, progression-free probability (PFP) after radical prostatectomy (Fig. 15.7).

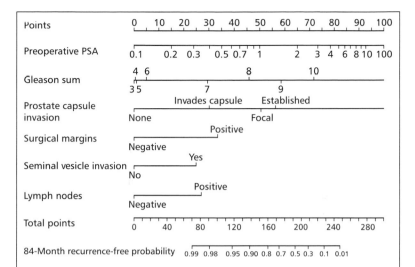

Instructions for physician
Locate the patient's PSA on the **PSA** axis. Draw a straight line upwards to the **Points** axis to determine how many points towards recurrence the patient receives for his PSA. Repeat this process for the other axes, each time drawing straight upward to the **Points** axis. Sum the points achieved for each predictor and locate this sum on the **Total Points** axis. Draw a line straight down to find the patient's probability of remaining recurrence free for 84 months assuming he does not die of another cause first.

Instruction to patient
'Mr X, if we had 100 men exactly like you, we would expect between *<predicted percentage from nomogram – 10%>* and *<predicted percentage + 10%>* to remain free of their disease at 7 years following radical prostatectomy, and recurrence after 7 years is very rare.'

Fig. 15.7 Postoperative nomogram estimating the likelihood of prostate cancer recurrence, based on data from 996 patients treated at the Methodist Hospital, Houston, Texas. [From: Kattan MW et al, *J Clin Oncol* **117**: 1499–1507, 1999]

[Kattan MW, *J Clin Oncol* **17**: 1499–1507, 1999]
[Stephenson AJ, *J Clin Oncol* **23**: 7005–7012, 2005]
– These nomograms have recently been validated using CaPSURE. [Greene KL, *J Urol* **171**: 2255–2259, 2004]

• Other pretreatment variables that are currently being studied include:
  1. The number and percentage of (+) biopsy cores.

2. The percentage of high-grade cancer in the biopsy specimen.
3. Microvessel density and DNA ploidy.
4. Additional molecular tumor markers (i.e. hyaluronidase and hyaluronic acid, $p53$, etc.).
5. Endorectal magnetic resonance imaging findings.
6. The percentage of prostate cancer relative to benign prostate in the final pathologic specimen.

Complications

- Complications of radical prostatectomy can be categorized as perioperative and late complications.

- Perioperative complications and their relative frequency from several series are summarized in Table 15.2.

- Late complications of radical prostatectomy include strictures of the vesicourethral anastomosis, changes in health-related quality of life, and persistent sexual and urinary dysfunction.

- Using Surveillance, Epidemiology, and End Results (SEER) Data.
  - Medicare-linked database to evaluate outcome data in 11,522 patients who underwent radical prostatectomy between 1992 and 1996.
  - RESULTS:
    - Perioperative complications and late urinary complications (incontinence, bladder-neck obstruction, and urethral strictures) → significantly ↓ when the operation was performed in a high-volume hospital by a surgeon who performed a large number of radical prostatectomies.
    [Begg CB, *N Engl J Med* **346**(15): 1138–1144, 2002]

- In addition to contributing to a ↓ mortality associated with radical prostatectomy, hospital volumes also seem to correlate with a ↓ postoperative length of stay and overall hospital charges.
  [Ellison LM, *J Urol* **163**: 867–869, 2000]
- In a series of 3,477 consecutive radical prostatectomies performed by one surgeon, the overall complication rate of radical prostatectomy ↓ significantly between the pre-PSA-screening era (16.9% in 1983–1991) and the post-PSA-screening era (7.4% in 1992–2003).
  - In this study, the rate of postoperative anastomotic strictures ↓ from 8% to 1.5%, which was speculated to be a result of an ↑ in the size of the lumen of the bladder neck from 18-French to 22- or 24-French.

Table 15.2 Perioperative morbidity and mortality in several contemporary series of radical prostatectomy patients

Series	No. of patients	Overall	Death	Thrombo-embolic	Cardio-vascular	Wound injury	Rectal	Lymphocele
[Kundu K, J Urol 172: 2227–2231, 2004]	3,477	32C (9)	0	45 (1.3)	3 (0.1)	26 (0.7)	NS	7 (0.2)
[Dilliogluglil O, J Urol 157: 1760–1767, 1997]	472	46 (9.8)	2 (0.4)	6 (1.3)	14 (3)	13 (2.9)	3 (0.6)	5 (1.1)
[Maffezzini M, Urology 61: 982–986, 2003]	300	19 (6.3)	0	1 (0.3)	NS	2 (0.7)	1 (0.3)	3 (1)
[Lepor H, Urology 62: 702–706, 2003]	500	26 (5.2)	0	0	3 (0.6)	6 (1.2)	0	0
[Rassweiler J, J Urol 169: 1689–1693, 2003]	219	40 (18.2)	1 (0.5)	5 (2.3)	0	5 (2.3)	3 (1.4)	15 (6.9)
[Chang SS, Cancer 104: 747–751, 2005]	994	44 (7.2)	0	1 (0.1)	1 (0.1)	4 (0.4)	0	0

Perioperative complications

Mortality

- Perioperative mortality following radical prostatectomy is approximately 0.5%.

- A review of the mortality data of 11,010 radical prostatectomies performed over a 10-year period in Canada demonstrated that the 30-day mortality was associated with older patient age, an antecedent history of either cardiovascular disease or stroke, and having had surgery in the earlier years of the review.
  [Alibhai SMH, *J Natl Cancer Inst* **97**(20): 1525–1532, 2005]

- In a study of 66,232 radical prostatectomies performed in the USA, mortality declined from 0.3% to 0.17% when the surgery was performed in hospital centers that perform a higher volume of these procedures.
  [Ellison LM, *J Urol* **163**: 867–869, 2000]

- We have reported only one perioperative death (0.07%) in more than 1,364 radical prostatectomies performed by a single surgeon.
  [Koya MP, *BJU Int* **96**(7): 1019–1021, 2005]

Hemorrhage

- The average blood loss during radical prostatectomy varies, with most centers reporting losses of 300–1000 ml.

- The literature supports the observation that the average transfusion rate in patients undergoing radical prostatectomy has ↓ significantly over the last several years, with 4.5–10% of patients receiving allogenic transfusions.
  [Goad JR, *J Urol* **154**: 2103–2109, 1995]
  [Chang SS, *J Urol* **171**(5): 1861–1865, 2004]
  [Farham SB, *Urology* **67**(2): 360–363, 2006]

- Some of the factors related to the declining need for allogenic blood transfusion include: experience of the surgeon, the use of preoperative autologous blood donation, and the intraoperative use of a cell saver.
  [Goodnough LM, *Urology* **44**: 226–231, 1994]
  [Nieder AM, *Urology* **65**(4): 730–734, 2005]
  - We have advocated intraoperative use of a cell saver, which has been found to be safe and has not been associated with a higher PSA recurrence rate than would be expected in our patients based on their pathologic features.

- Preoperative use of erythropoietin is another technique that has been advocated for minimizing the transfusion risk in the radical prostatectomy patient.
  [Rosenblum N, J Urol **163**: 829–833, 2000]

Rectal and ureteral injuries

- Rectal injury during radical prostatectomy occurs in < 1% of patients.

- Prior radiation therapy, a history of antecedent rectal surgery, or a prior transurethral resection of the prostate (TURP) may ↑ the risk of a rectal injury at the time of radical prostatectomy.
  [McLaren RH, *Urology* **42**: 401–405, 1993]

- It is a potentially serious complication that can lead to a rectourethral fistula, especially if not recognized intraoperatively.

- A mechanical bowel preparation or a Fleets enema administered the evening prior to surgery has been advocated in order to enhance the safety of a primary rectal closure, in the event of an intraoperative rectal injury.

- Following complete removal of the prostate, a two-layered closure of the injured rectal wall with dilatation of the anal sphincter should be performed.
  - In addition, interposition of a segment of omentum between the rectum and vesicourethral anastomosis has been described in order to ↓ the risk of fistula formation.
    [Borland RN, J Urol **147**: 905–907, 1992]

- Ureteral injuries are extremely rare, and usually occur when dissecting the base of the prostate off the bladder or during dissection of the seminal vesicles.
  - An intraoperative knowledge of where the ureteral orifices are situated prior to transection of the posterior bladder neck, and during tennis-racquet closure of the bladder neck, is important in avoiding these injuries.
  - If a ureteral transection injury is recognized, it requires a formal ureteral reimplantation.

Medical complications of radical prostatectomy

- A variety of perioperative medical complications may occur in patients undergoing radical prostatectomy.

- These include cardiac as well as thromboembolic complications.
  - While the incidence of these individual complications is relatively low, the surgeon should have an appreciation and awareness of the associated risk factors.

- Because of the potential risk of rapid blood loss associated with this procedure, we recommend a low threshold for a full cardiology evaluation of these ♂, particularly those who have risk factors for underlying heart disease (age > 65 years, documented history of coronary artery disease).

- Appropriate medical clearance should be obtained prior to surgery, particularly for those ♂ with a family history of heart disease, hypertension, or diabetes.

- The perioperative use of beta blockers for select individuals should be addressed, and may provide additional safety in patients undergoing non-cardiac surgery.
  [Lindenauer PK, *N Engl J Med* **353**(4): 349–361, 2005]

- The risk of deep vein thrombosis and subsequent pulmonary embolus → 1–3% of patients undergoing radical prostatectomy.
  - Recent data have shown a ↓ in the incidence of perioperative thromboembolic events in some series.
    [Catalona WJ, *J Urol* **162**: 433–438, 1999]
    [Lepor H, *J Urol* **166**: 1729–1733, 2001]
  - In a consecutive series of 1,364 patients undergoing radical prostatectomy from our center, there were only 3 (0.25%) venous thromboembolic events, and no patient had a pulmonary embolus.
    [Koya MP, *BJU Int* **96**(7): 1019–1021, 2005]
    - This is likely a result of diminished surgery times, earlier ambulation following surgery, and the use of sequential pneumatic compression stockings, which are applied prior to the induction of anesthesia.
  - Postoperative use of heparin may ↓ the incidence of perioperative thromboembolic occurrences; however, it may also be associated with an ↑ risk of bleeding and prolonged lymphatic drainage.
    [Keech DW, *AUA Update Series* **13**: Lesson 6, 1994]
    - We do not utilize perioperative anticoagulation therapy routinely in patients undergoing radical prostatectomy.

Lymphocele

- Performance of a modified pelvic lymphadenectomy rarely results in a lymphocele.

- Symptomatic lymphoceles require percutaneous drainage, with the use of a sclerosing agent, if the lymphocele does not resolve within a short period of time.

- Laparoscopic or open marsupialization of the lymphocele into the peritoneal cavity may be done for recurrent lymphoceles.

Persistent urinary extravasation from the anastomosis

- Persistent postoperative urinary extravasation from the anastomosis is a rare event following radical prostatectomy.
  - The integrity of the vesicourethral anastomosis should be tested prior to closure by administering saline into the Foley catheter after all the anastomotic sutures have been tied.
  - The majority of patients have the drain removed by the first or second postoperative day, if it is even placed in the first place.
  - If there is persistent drainage of > 50–75 ml per shift, a blood urea nitrogen (BUN) and creatinine level from the drainage fluid is used to differentiate a urinary fistula from a lymphatic leak.

- Even large amounts of urinary drainage into the closed suction drain almost always resolve spontaneously.
  - Provided that the catheter is in a good position.
  - If there is any suspicion that the catheter has become dislodged, a ureteral injury was incurred at the time of the prostatectomy, or if the drain is too close to the anastomosis, a formal evaluation may be initiated.
    - This includes a cystogram, and possible computerized tomography (CT) urogram.
  - Management of these complications may require surgical intervention; however, this is a rare event in the literature.

Late complications

Anastomotic strictures

- Strictures of the vesicourethral anastomosis occur in 0.7–16% of radical prostatectomies.
  - Anastomotic strictures may present with a variety of symptoms, including:
    - ↓ caliber of the urinary stream, frank urinary retention, or worsening urinary incontinence following radical prostatectomy.
    - Many strictures are likely asymptomatic as well.
  - The etiology for strictures of the anastomosis is speculative.

- Theories for the occurrence of these strictures include:
  - The presence of a perianastomotic hematoma, ischemia of the bladder neck and urethra, and overzealous narrowing of the bladder neck during the tennis-racquet closure.
- Treatment varies depending on the severity of the stricture, and includes:
  - Dilatation, dilatation with instillation of steroids, and
  - Transurethral incision of the bladder neck.

Changes in quality of life measures

- The assessment of health-related quality of life (HRQOL) following radical prostatectomy requires an evaluation of both general and disease-specific issues facing the prostate cancer patient.

- General HRQOL domains include one's sense of overall well-being and function in the physical, emotional, and social domains.

- Prostate-cancer-specific HRQOL domains following radical prostatectomy include urinary and sexual function.
  [Penson DF, AUA *Update Series* **XX**: Lesson 3, 18022, 1999]

- It is well recognized that physicians grossly underestimate the impact of changes in a variety of quality-of-life issues facing the radical prostatectomy patient.
  [Litwin M, *J Urol* **159**: 1988–1992, 1998]
  - Therefore, assessment of HRQOL issues is best performed using self-administered, validated questionnaires.

- Utilizing these validated instruments to assess the general HRQOL following radical prostatectomy, several studies have noted relatively few changes in general HRQOL compared with:
  - Age-matched, ZIP-code-matched controls.
    [Litwin MS, *JAMA* **273**(2): 129–135, 1995]
  - ♂ undergoing transurethral prostatectomy for benign disease.
    [Fowler FJ, *Urology* **45**(6): 1007–1011, 1995]
  - Age- and sex-adjusted Dutch population data.
    [Madalinska JB, *J Clin Oncol* **19**(6): 1619–1628, 2001]
  - Groups of otherwise healthy ♂ volunteers.
    [Wei JT, *J Clin Oncol* **20**: 557–566, 2002]

- While the overall general HRQOL scores may initially decline immediately following surgery, one study demonstrated a significant improvement back to baseline after the first year.
  [Lubek DP, *Urology* **53**(1): 180–186, 1999]

- More recently, studies have observed some subtle differences in the overall HRQOL in patients with localized prostate cancer, possibly reflecting the effects of stage migration and younger patients detected in screened populations.
    - In a comparison of 783 untreated ♂ with incidental prostate cancer with 1,928 age-matched healthy controls, ♂ with prostate cancer had significantly better physical function and less bodily pain than controls, but had worse general health, vitality, social function, and role limitations as a result of physical and emotional problems.
    [Bacon CG, *Cancer* **94**: 862–871, 2002]
    - This suggests that the disease itself, and not only the treatment, may impact HRQOL.

- The initial impact of altered sexual and urinary function on overall HRQOL has been well documented.

- Using several validated instruments, one study demonstrated that post-prostatectomy erectile dysfunction correlated positively with vigor and negatively with incontinence and depression.
[Lim AJ, *J Urol* **154**(4): 1420–1425, 1995]
    - In this same study, urinary incontinence positively correlated with tension, fatigue, and depression, and inversely correlated with vigor and social well-being.

- Despite this, several studies have shown that, although radical prostatectomy is known to have an effect on potency and continence, it appears to have little, if any, effect on long-term general HRQOL.
[Penson DF, *AUA Update Series* **XX**: Lesson 3, 18022, 1999]

Prostate-cancer-specific HRQOL

Sexual function

- Erectile dysfunction is defined as the persistent inability to achieve or maintain an erection of sufficient rigidity and duration for satisfactory sexual relations.
[National Institutes of Health, *NIH Consensus Statement: Impotence* **10**(4): 1992]

- Overall, 50% of ♂ aged 40–70 years have varying degrees of erectile dysfunction.
[Feldman HA, *J Urol* **151**(1): 54–61, 1994]

- Risk factors besides age include hypertension, diabetes mellitus, cardiovascular disease, dyslipidemia, and depression.

- Prior to the advent of the anatomical nerve-sparing radical prostatectomy, virtually all patients undergoing this surgery had erectile dysfunction.

- Early published radical prostatectomy series found that age, preoperative potency, the number of neurovascular bundles preserved, and final pathologic stage all influenced the preservation of erectile function in ♂ undergoing prostate cancer surgery.
  [Quinlan DM, *J Urol* **145**(5): 998–1002, 1991]
  [Catalona WJ, *J Urol* **143**: 538–543, 1990]

- While the published potency preservation rates in these series varied between 63% and 76%, another study demonstrated that only half of those patients reporting erections following prostatectomy were actually able to have sexual intercourse.
  [Geary ES, *J Urol* **154**: 145–149, 1995]

- Studies that have utilized self-administered instruments have found that 21–50% of patients can have erections firm enough for intercourse following radical prostatectomy.
  [Talcott JA, *J Natl Cancer Inst* **89**(55): 1117–1123, 1997]
  [Stanford JL, *JAMA* **283**(3): 354–360, 2000]
  [Noldus J, *Eur Urol* **142**(2): 118–124, 2002]

- In addition, the return of potency following radical prostatectomy has been found to be a time-dependent process, in which there is a gradual return of potency in many individuals during the first 24 months.
  [Litwin MS, *Urology* **54**(3): 503–508, 1999]
  [Stanford JL, *JAMA* **283**(3): 354–360, 2000]

- The advent of the phosphodiesterase type-5 (PDE-5) agents has significantly impacted many ♂ with post-prostatectomy erectile dysfunction.
  - PDE-5 inhibitors are the first line of therapy in the management of erectile dysfunction in ♂ who have undergone nerve-sparing radical prostatectomy.
  - Improvements in frequency of penetration, the ability to maintain an erection, and both patient and spousal satisfaction are seen in up to 70% of cases.
    [Zippe CD, *Urology* **52**(6): 963–966, 1998]
  - For those ♂ who do not respond to PDE-5 inhibitors, intracavernous injection therapy, transurethral therapy, vacuum erection devices, and implantation of a penile prosthesis are additional options.
    - Use of these adjunctive therapies is discussed in a recent review of management strategies to use when PDE-5 inhibitors fail.
      [Kava BR, *Rev Urol* **7**(Suppl 2): S29–S50, 2005]

Urinary dysfunction

- The International Continence Society defines continence as the involuntary loss of urine, which is a social or hygiene problem that is objectively demonstrable.
  [Abrams P, *Urology* **61**(1): 37–49, 2003]

- The number of pads used by an individual following radical prostatectomy has been used as a convenient endpoint in determining outcome success following radical prostatectomy.

- Using these criteria, two recent large series have demonstrated continence rates between 91% and 95% between 18 and 24 months following radical prostatectomy.
  [Catalona WJ, *J Urol* **162**: 433–438, 1999]
  [Bianco FJ, *Urology* **66**(Suppl 5A): 83–94, 2005]
  - In the first of these series, continence (defined as no need for any pad for protection) was only found to be higher in younger ♂, and was independent of nerve preservation, clinical stage, pathologic stage, postoperative radiation therapy, or the number of prior prostatectomies performed by the surgeon.

- The number of pads used per day is a convenient measure, but when used alone provides a poor assessment of voiding dysfunction following radical prostatectomy.

- Similar to the data from CaPSURE for erectile dysfunction, physicians once again underestimate the reduction in HRQOL imposed by urinary incontinence.
  [Litwin M, *J Urol* **159**: 1988–1992, 1998]

- Self-administered, validated questionnaires should be used to derive a meaningful estimate of:
  1. The type and degree of urinary dysfunction.
  2. The level of dysfunction and the degree of bother experienced by the patient.
  3. The disease-specific and general domains of the HRQOL.
     [Penson DF, *AUA Update Series* **XX**: Lesson 3, 18022, 1999]

- Several recent series have reported on postoperative continence in patients using such instruments.

- One of these was the prostate cancer outcomes study, which has recently reported 5-year data on a sample population of 1,288 ♂ from one of six SEER registries in the USA.
  [Penson DF, *J Urol* **173**: 1701–1705, 2005]

- RESULTS:
  - 25% of ♂ reported frequent urination or lack of urinary control at 6 months.
  - By 24 months, the proportion of ♂ reporting this much leakage had ↓ to 10.4%, and by 5 years it was 13.9%.
  - Interestingly, 40% of ♂ at 6 months and 22% of ♂ at 5 years still reported using 1–2 pads/day.
    - Yet, 11% and 13% of ♂ at 2 and 5 years, respectively, considered urinary incontinence a moderate or great problem.

- In another study, 342 patients undergoing radical prostatectomy were prospectively evaluated using the UCLA Prostate Cancer Index. [Haffner MC, *Urology* **66**: 371–376, 2005]
  - This confirmed that the 24-month actuarial likelihood of returning to baseline urinary function and bother was 92% or greater, irrespective of the nerve-sparing status.

- A study was done in a large, managed-care population in California. [Litwin MS, JAMA **273**(2): 129–135, 1995]
  - RESULTS:
    - 40% of patients had daily leakage of urine.
    - 90% of patients used ≤ 2 pads/day.
    - 30% claimed total urinary control.
    - 45% considered their problem to be occasional.

Summary

- Over the last 25 years dramatic improvements have been made in our ability to perform radical prostatectomy.

- With ♂ being diagnosed with prostate cancer at an earlier stage and at a younger age, radical prostatectomy will certainly maintain a leading role in the treatment of this disease in the future.

- At this time, a variety of techniques for performing radical prostatectomy using laparoscopic techniques are currently being utilized. These will likely play an increasing role in the future.

- Nevertheless, a sound understanding of the technical components of open radical prostatectomy, as well as its ability to provide oncologic control and minimize adverse effects on HRQOL, and sexual and urinary function, is necessary in order to provide a standard against which future treatment modifications will be compared.

16

Post-prostatectomy radiation therapy

- Patients with tumor confined within the prostate at prostatectomy (pT_2 disease) who also have (–) margins have an 84–98% long-term progression-free survival (PFS) compared to a 37–70% PFS in patients with extraprostatic extension (pT_3) disease after prostatectomy.

- Prostate-specific antigen (PSA) velocity < 0.75 ng/ml per year is seen in patients with isolated local recurrence.
  [Partin AW, *Urology* **43**: 649–659, 1994]
  - Later recurrences, beyond 1 year, have a greater chance of having isolated local recurrences and are thus more amenable to treatment with radiation.

Adjuvant post-prostatectomy radiation therapy

- Adjuvant post-prostatectomy radiation is delivered in the immediate post-prostatectomy period based on adverse pathologic features.

- Advantage: earlier treatment of a smaller tumor volume.

- Postoperative radiation ↑ local control, but not survival.
  [Schild S, *Mayo Clin Proc* **69**: 613–619, 1994]
  [Wu JJ, *Int J Radiat Oncol Biol Phys* **32**: 317–323, 1995]
  [Anscher MS, *Int J Radiat Oncol Biol Phys* **33**: 37–43, 1995]

Prospective randomized trials

- European Organisation for Research and Treatment of Cancer (EORTC) 2291.

[Bolla M, *Lancet* **366**(9485): 572–578, 2005]
- A phase III, randomized study in 1005 patients with T_0–T_3 and pT_2–T_3 prostate adenocarcinoma who were post-prostatectomy with one or more pathologic risk factors (capsule perforation, (+) surgical margins, invasion of seminal vesicles).
  - Group I: no radiation was given initially (i.e. wait and see policy); if salvaged with radiation, 70 Gy were given.
  - Group II: 60 Gy of radiation was given within 16 weeks after surgery (50 Gy included prostate and seminal vesicle bed, and final 10 Gy boost included the prostate bed alone).
- Median follow-up → 5 years.
- RESULTS:
  - Biochemical PFS was significantly better in the irradiated group (74% vs 52.6%, $p = 0.0001$).
  - Clinical PFS was significantly better in the irradiated group ($p = 0.0009$).
  - Cumulative rate of locoregional failure at 5 years was significantly lower in the irradiated group (5.4% vs 15.4%, $p<0.0001$).
- SIDE-EFFECTS:
  - There were more grade 2 or 3 toxicities in the postoperative radiation group ($p = 0.0005$).
  - The rate of grade 3 or higher toxicity was 2.6% in the watch-and-wait group vs 4.2% in the postoperative radiation group at 5 years.
- CONCLUSIONS:
  - Immediate external beam radiation after radical prostatectomy improves biochemical PFS and local control in patients with (+) margins, or pT_3 disease.
- LIMITATIONS OF THE STUDY:
  - Gleason grade not assessed.
  - Only WHO criteria were assessed.
  - No central pathology review was done.
  - No comparison with early salvage (before 1 ng/ml); 34.4% of those who received salvage therapy had locoregional clinical progression.

- Southwest Oncology Group (SWOG) 8794.
  [Swanson, GP, *Int J Radiat Oncol Biol Phys* **63**(1 Suppl 1): S1, 2005]
  - 473 patients with extracapsular extension, (+) margins and/or seminal vesicle involvement after prostatectomy were randomized.
    - Group I: radiation (60–64 Gy).
    - Group II: observation.

- Median follow-up → 9.7 years.
- RESULTS:
  - Biochemical disease-free survival (PSA < 0.4 ng/ml) was significantly improved in the radiation vs observation group: 61% vs 38% and 47% vs 23% at 5 and 10 years, respectively.
  - Metastases-free survival and overall survival improved but did not achieve statistical significance.
- SIDE-EFFECTS (genitourinary and gastrointestinal):
  - Were greater in the radiation group at 6 weeks during the radiation, but by 2 years there was no significant difference in quality (QOL) of life between the two groups.
- CONCLUSIONS:
  - Adjuvant radiation for pT_3 disease improves 5- and 10-year disease-free survival but not overall or metastases-free survival.
  - Radiation prevented the need for androgen ablation in some patients and delayed the use by 2.5 years in the rest.
  - Long-term QOL was not adversely affected by radiation.
  - Pathologic T_3 patients should be offered postoperative radiation.

Salvage post-prostatectomy radiation therapy after relapse

- The half-life of PSA is 3.2 days; PSA should fall to undetectable levels by 3–4 weeks after surgery.
  [Oesterling JE, *J Urol* **139**: 766–772, 1988]

- Undetectable levels depend on the assay, but if levels are > 0.1 ng/ml there is a high likelihood of subsequent biochemical failure.
  [Vessella RL, *Urol Clin North Am* **20**: 607–619, 1993]

- Salvage treatment for biochemical persistent disease or relapsed disease.

- Up to half of patients with biochemical recurrence after prostatectomy have local recurrence, with the remainder having distant metastases alone or in combination with local recurrence.
  [Partin AW, *J Urol* **152**: 1358, 1994]

- Advantage: avoidance of unnecessary treatment of the 50% of patients who, although left with a (+) margin post-prostatectomy, will not relapse.

- The number of (+) margins may predict an ↑ likelihood of recurrence.
  - Patients with a single (+) margin may be followed and then treated with salvage radiation if there is recurrence.

- Patients with multiple (+) margins may be better served with adjuvant radiation.
  [Grossfield G, J Urol 164: 93–99, 2000]
- The PSA level at salvage predicts success.
  [Schild S, J Urol 156: 1725, 1996]
  - Salvage should be started at PSA ≤ 1 ng/ml.
  - Although levels of ≤ 2 ng/ml have also been shown to predict improved disease-free survival.
    [Foreman J, Int J Radiat Oncol Biol Phys 12: 185, 1986]
- Outcomes between adjuvant and salvage radiation are equivalent when salvage radiotherapy is initiated with a low PSA (< 1 ng/ml).
  [Nudell DM, Urology 54: 1049, 1999]
- American Society for Therapeutic Radiology and Oncology (ASTRO) consensus panel.
  [ASTRO Consensus Panel, J Clin Oncol 17: 1155–1163, 1999]
  - Consensus statements on radiation therapy of prostate cancer: guidelines for prostate re-biopsy after radiation and radiation therapy with rising PSA after radical prostatectomy.
  - Findings: waiting for secure evidence of biochemical failure (a PSA ↑ to 0.05 ng/ml) does not reduce the chances of successful salvage radiation; better results are obtained when treatment is initiated before a PSA threshold of 1.5 ng/ml.

Choice of postoperative versus salvage radiation

- Immediate/postoperative radiation if high risk, with seminal vesicle involvement, Gleason score ≥ 7, and multiple (+) margins.
- Salvage radiation in other patients as long as radiation is started early, when PSA is still < 1 ng/ml.
  [Nuddell DM, Urology 54: 1049–1057, 1999]

Radiation therapy techniques

- Dose.
  [Valicenti RK, Int J Radiat Oncol Biol Phys 42: 501–506, 1998]
  - Retrospective study of 86 patients with pathologic T_3N_0 adenocarcinoma of the prostate who received post-prostatectomy radiation therapy to the prostate and seminal vesicle bed to doses in the range 55.8–70.2 Gy (median 64.8 Gy).
    - Group I: 52 patients with an undetectable pre-irradiation PSA.

- Group II: 21 patients with PSA levels > 0.02 but < 2 ng/ml.
- RESULTS:
  - 3-year biochemical disease-free survival rates for group I were 91% and 57% for those receiving ≥ 61.5 Gy vs those receiving lower doses.
  - 3 year biochemical disease-free survival rates for group II were 79% and 33% for those receiving ≥ 64.8 Gy vs those receiving lower doses.
- CONCLUSION:
  - Postoperative doses of ≥ 64.8 Gy should be considered.

- Technique:
  - Pelvic radiation to the level of the bifurcation of the common iliac artery if Gleason score ≥ 7, seminal vesicle involvement, or (+) pelvic nodes.
    - This is followed by a boost to the prostate bed using three-dimensional (3D) conformal radiation therapy.
  - Low-risk patients can receive 3D conformal fields from the beginning. [Connolly J, *Urology* 47: 225–231, 1996]
    - Some authors recommend small fields to the bed from the start because the most common areas of recurrence (peri-anastomotic region (66%), retrovesical space (13%), bladder neck (16%)) would be included in the small field.

Morbidity of postoperative radiation

- Compared 95 irradiated and 293 non-irradiated patients post-prostatectomy.
  [Freeman JA, *J Urol* 149: 1029–1034, 1993]
  - RESULTS:
    - Continence/mild stress incontinence in 88% of non-irradiated and 87% of irradiated patients.
    - No urethral strictures seen in either group.
    - ↓ potency rates from 46% in non-irradiated to 18% in irradiated patients.

- Other groups also report complications, including grade 1 or 2 rectal bleeding (0–12%).

Role of hormone therapy with postoperative radiation

- Radiation Therapy Oncology Group (RTOG) 85-31.
  [Corn BW, *Urology* 54: 495–502, 1999]

- Subset analysis.
- 139 ♂ post-prostatectomy with high-risk features (capsular pene-tration and seminal vesicle involvement) who presented for adjuvant radiation treatment (60–65 Gy).
  - Group I: 79 ♂ who received radiation and immediate androgen ablation (the luteinizing hormone releasing hormone (LHRH) agonist goserelin 3.6 mg to start, during the last week of the radiation).
  - Group II: 68 ♂ who received radiation alone, with hormone ablation at relapse.
- RESULTS:
  - Freedom from biochemical relapse (< 0.5 ng/ml) at 5 years was 65% vs 42%.
  - On multivariate analysis, the use of radiation + immediate hormones was an independent factor predictive of freedom from biochemical failure.
- CONCLUSIONS:
  - Hormone ablation may be beneficial in this setting in con-junction with radiation.
- LIMITATION OF STUDY:
  - A subset analysis: the study was not designed to investigate this.

Other prospective studies, with pending results, of the benefit of adding hormonal ablation to radiation

- RTOG 0011.
  - High-risk patients (i.e. Gleason score ≥ 7, with capsular penetration, (+) margins, or seminal vesicle invasion) with a PSA < 0.2 ng/ml.
  - The study will determine whether the addition of androgen ablat-ion to radiation (63–66 Gy) is better than either alone.

- RTOG 96-01.
  - Patients with pT_2–pT_3 and/or (+) margins with ↑ PSA between 0.2 and 4 ng/ml who receive 64.8 Gy of radiation and are random-ized to either bicalutamide 150 mg/day or placebo for 2 years.

Cryotherapy for prostate cancer

History

[Shiohara K, *Urol Clin North Am* **30**: 725–736, 2003]
[Loening S, *Prostate* **1**(3): 279–286, 1980]
[*Stedman's Medical Dictionary*, 26th edn. Lippincott Williams & Wilkins, Baltimore, OH, 1995, p. 416]

- Cryotherapy is defined as the use of cold in the treatment of disease.

- Cryoablation is the destruction of tissue by local induction of extremely cold temperatures.

- Modern cryotherapy began in 1966 with closed circulation liquid nitrogen probes.

- The first transurethral cryoablation of prostate tissue was in 1966 for benign hypertrophy.

- Cryoablation was first used to treat cancer of the prostate in 1968 via an open transperineal approach; the percutaneous approach was first conducted in 1974.

- Advances in the last 15 years in the use of cryotherapy for prostate cancer include:
  - Freezing mechanisms – argon gas rather than liquid nitrogen.
  - Simultaneous use of multiple cryoprobes, and smaller diameter of gas-containing probes vs liquid-containing probes.
  - Standard use of warming catheter per urethra.
  - Real-time transrectal ultrasound scanning to monitor freezing and probe placement.

- Use of cryotherapy for prostate cancer is not common in urologic practice.
  - 1.25% of patients diagnosed with localized prostate cancer since 1997 received cryotherapy as the primary treatment.

Cryobiology

[Baust JG, *Cryobiology* **48**(2): 190–204, 2004]
[Tatsutani K, *Urology* **48**: 441–447, 1996]
[Gage AA, *Cryobiology* **15**: 415–425, 1978]
[Mazur P, *Science* **168**: 939–949, 1970]

- Freezing mechanism.
  - The freezing medium is compressed liquid nitrogen or argon.
  - The freezing medium is administered locally to the gland via probes inserted in the prostate gland under ultrasound guidance.
  - The medium is delivered through a thin central lumen, and partially evaporated gas returns to the base of the probe via an outer chamber that is in intimate contact with the tissue to be destroyed.
  - The gas begins to expand as it evaporates because of its exposure to body temperature.
  - The Joule–Thompson principle states that an expanding gas will draw heat from its surroundings into the circulating gas.

- Mechanism of tissue destruction.
  - Extracellular fluid crystallizes when frozen to temperatures $< 0°C$. This causes an $\uparrow$ in the extracellular osmotic pressure, a shift of water from the intracellular space, and cell dehydration.
  - Electrolyte changes within the cell cause a drop in pH, with subsequent denaturing of intracellular proteins.
  - Intracellular fluid crystallizes, which results in cell membrane injury.
  - Thawing results in a rapid shift of fluid back into the intracellular space, and subsequent cell lysis.
  - Freezing of the vasculature results in microthrombi, which cause local tissue ischemia.

- Tissue ablation factors.
  - The lowest temperature achieved should be, at most, $-40°C$.
  - The velocity of cooling is an important predictor of cell death. Faster rates of freezing are associated with increased cell destruction.
  - Slower thawing is associated with more effective cell destruction.
  - Multiple freeze–thaw cycles are important in expanding zones of necrosis. Two tissue zones exist in cryoablation: a central zone of

necrosis and a peripheral zone of injury. This is seen on an ultrasound scan as an ice ball. The central zone of necrosis increases considerably with a second freeze–thaw cycle as opposed to a single cycle.
- Heat sinks are defined as areas of hypervascularity that may not achieve target temperatures throughout the area of treatment.

- Equipment for performing cryotherapy.
  - Cryosurgical devices available in the USA use either liquid nitrogen or argon.
  - Probe diameters vary in the range 1.5–2.4 mm. A larger probe diameter results in a wider diameter ice ball, but less probes can be placed. All cryoprobes have a similar double-lumen structure.
  - A urethral warming catheter is always used to protect the urethra and external sphincter mechanism from the damaging effects of cooling. It is a closed double-lumen catheter with continuously circulating saline heated to 38–40°C.

- Cryotherapy has been used either as primary therapy, or salvage therapy following prior radiation or cryotherapy, for prostate cancer

Patient selection for primary treatment of prostate cancer

[Johnson DB, *J Endourol* **17**(8): 627–632, 2003]
[Shiohara K, *Urol Clin North Am* **30**: 725–736, 2003]
[Pisters LL, *J Urol* **157**(3): 921–925, 1997]

- Any patient with clinically localized prostate cancer, with a prostate-specific antigen (PSA) level < 10 ng/ml, clinical stage T_{1c} or T_{2a}, a Gleason sum of ≤ 6, and who has a life expectancy of at least 10 years with regard to other variables outside cancer, is a good candidate for cryotherapy as primary treatment.

- Those with a higher Gleason score or preoperative PSA are at increased risk of extracapsular extension, and thus would not be cured.

- Patients who are interested in preservation of erectile function are best suited to an alternative therapy, as impotency rates are higher for cryotherapy than for other forms of local treatment.

- Prostate glands > 50 cm³ are difficult to treat by cryotherapy because complete gland ablation may not be feasible. No formal studies comment on the use of neoadjuvant hormone therapy to reduce gland size, but several authors suggest this for larger glands.

- Other contraindications to cryotherapy include:
  - Prior abdominoperineal resection of the rectum.
  - Rectal inflammatory disease.
  - Anal stricture.
  - History of transurethral resection of the prostate.

- Cryoablation has also been used effectively as salvage therapy after radiation treatment.

Cancer-related outcomes after cryosurgical ablation of the prostate

- [Long JP, *Urology* **57**: 518–523, 2001]
  - 5-year retrospective, multi-institutional analysis of 975 patients who underwent cryoablation of the prostate as primary therapy.
  - Patients were stratified into three risk groups.
    - Low risk: stage T_{2a} or lower, PSA ≤ 10 ng/ml, Gleason score ≤ 6.
    - Moderate risk (one of the following risk factors): stage T_{2b} or higher, PSA > 10 ng/ml, or Gleason score ≥ 7.
    - High risk: 2 or 3 of the above risk factors.
  - Median follow-up: 24 months.
  - RESULTS:
    - % of patients with biochemical-free survival (set at PSA < 1.0 ng/ml):
      - Low risk: 76%.
      - Moderate risk: 61%.
      - High risk: 36%.
    - These results were compared to those in patients who underwent radiation therapy who were also stratified according to the three risk groups.
  - CONCLUSIONS:
    - The rates of biochemical-free survival are comparable to those seen with treatment by radiotherapy.
  - LIMITATION OF THE STUDY:
    - Retrospective, so proper comparison with radiotherapy in a prospective, randomized fashion was not possible.

- [Shinohara K, *J Urol* **158**(6): 2206–2209, 1997]
  - 3-year, retrospective analysis of 134 patients who underwent cryoablative surgery for prostate cancer. Of these, 110 had adequate follow-up and did not receive adjuvant androgen deprivation. Neoadjuvant androgen blockade was provided to those patients with locally extensive cancer and those with a gland size ≥ 50 cm³.

Follow-up included PSA determination at 3, 6, and 12 months postoperatively, and then every 6 months thereafter. Prostate biopsy was performed at 6 months and/or when there was any evidence of failure (PSA nadir ≥ 0.5 ng/ml, or PSA elevation after nadir ≥ 0.2 ng/ml). Patients were grouped into one of three categories based on PSA nadir (< 0.1, 0.1–0.4, and ≥ 0.5 ng/ml).

- Mean follow-up: 17.6 months.
- RESULTS:
  - % of patients who experienced biochemical failure (rise in PSA of ≥ 0.2 ng/ml):
    - PSA nadir < 0.1 ng/ml: 21%.
    - PSA nadir 0.1–0.4 ng/ml: 48%.
    - PSA nadir > 0.5 ng/ml: these patients had either immediate local failure (46%), subsequent biochemical failure (43%), or an extremely high nadir.
  - % of patients who had a (+) biopsy:
    - PSA nadir < 0.1 ng/ml: 7%.
    - PSA nadir 0.1–0.4 ng/ml: 22%.
    - PSA nadir > 0.5 ng/ml: 60%.
- CONCLUSIONS:
  - PSA nadir ≤ 0.4 ng/ml should be achieved following cryotherapy. Higher values are associated with a significant risk of biochemical failure and residual disease on subsequent biopsy.
- LIMITATION OF THE STUDY:
  - Retrospective study with no comparison group or control group.

- [Cohen JK, *Urology* **47**(3): 395–401, 1996]
  - 2-year, retrospective analysis of 383 patients who underwent 448 cryotherapies for prostate cancer.
    - 'Virgin' group: 239 patients (followed for a minimum of 21 months and received no prior treatment).
    - 'ADT' group: 144 patients who had been on androgen deprivation prior to cryoablation.
  - Post-treatment biopsy and serum PSA were performed at 21–24 months.
  - RESULTS:
    - % of (–) biopsies from 114 patients at a minimum of 21 months post-treatment:
      - Virgin group: 79%.
      - ADT group: 88%.
    - % with PSA < 0.4 ng/ml from 163 patients at a minimum of 21 months post-treatment:

- – Virgin group: 60%.
- – ADT group: 40%.
- CONCLUSIONS:
  - – Cryosurgical ablation appears to be effective in obtaining local control, as measured by biopsy and serum PSA at ≥ 21 months post-treatment.
  - – These results compared favorably and seemed more effective than similar data obtained following radiation treatment.
- LIMITATION OF STUDY:
  - – Retrospective study with no comparison group or control group.

Cryosurgical ablation as salvage therapy after radiation treatment

- Some studies have shown efficacy of cryosurgery in the treatment of locally recurrent prostate cancer after radiation therapy (i.e. salvage cryotherapy).

- [Ghafar MA, J Urol **166**: 1333–1338, 2001]
  - Retrospective review of 38 ♂, mean age 71.9 years, who underwent salvage cryosurgery for locally recurrent disease after radiation. All had biochemical recurrence, which was defined as a rise in PSA of > 0.3 ng/ml from the nadir. Recurrent cancer was proven by subsequent prostate biopsy in all patients. Metastatic disease was ruled out prior to salvage therapy, and all patients received 3 months of neoadjuvant therapy prior to salvage.
  - RESULTS:
    - – 31 (81.5%) ♂ reached a PSA nadir of ≤ 0.1 ng/ml. Biochemical recurrence-free survival was 86% at 1 year and 74% at 2 years post-salvage treatment.
    - – Rates of urinary tract infection, urinary incontinence, and scrotal edema were 2.6%, 7.9%, and 10.5%, respectively. There was no reported incidence of rectourethral fistula, urethral sloughing, or urinary retention.
  - CONCLUSIONS:
    - – Cryosurgical ablation of the prostate used as salvage therapy post-radiation was safe and effective in this patient group.
  - LIMITATIONS OF THE STUDY:
    - – Retrospective study with no comparison group or control group.
    - – Small group of patients.

- [Izawa J, *J Urol* **165**: 867–870, 2001]
  - A retrospective analysis of 145 patients who underwent salvage cryosurgery after external beam radiation therapy. Of these, 107 underwent post-cryotherapy prostate biopsy. Numerous variables were then evaluated using univariate and multivariate analysis, the goal of which was to observe which variables would predict (+) biopsy after salvage therapy.
  - RESULTS:
    - Prostate biopsy was (+) in 23 (21%) of cases after salvage therapy.
    - On univariate analysis, predictors of a (+) biopsy (with statistical significance) included:
      - Higher initial stage.
      - Higher pre-cryotherapy PSA.
      - Number of (+) biopsy cores before salvage therapy.
      - Higher PSA nadir after salvage therapy.
      - Fewer cryoprobes and number of freeze–thaw cycles.
      - Negative history of androgen-deprivation therapy.
    - On multivariate analysis, predictors of (+) biopsy (with statistical significance) included:
      - Fewer cryoprobes used.
      - Higher post-cryotherapy PSA nadir.
  - CONCLUSIONS:
    - Patients with initial clinical stage T_2 or less and PSA < 10 ng/ml have a higher rate of (–) biopsy after salvage cryotherapy.
    - Detectable PSA after salvage therapy is a strong predictor of (+) biopsy, and thus local failure.
  - LIMITATION OF THE STUDY:
    - Retrospective study with no comparison group or control group.

- [Pisters LL, *J Urol* **157**(3): 921–925, 1997]
  - Phase I/II study of 150 patients with locally recurrent prostate cancer following radiation, hormone therapy, and/or systemic chemotherapy. 71 patients had a single freeze–thaw cycle as salvage cryoablation, and 79 had a double cycle. PSA was measured every 3 months postoperatively, and prostate biopsy was performed at 6 months.
  - Mean follow-up: those who underwent a single freeze–thaw cycle, 17.3 months; those who underwent a double cycle, 10 months.
  - RESULTS:
    - 45 (31%) patients had persistently undetectable PSA.
    - Of those who received radiation alone as primary therapy for prostate cancer:

- Those who had a single freeze–thaw cycle had a (–) biopsy rate of 71%.
- Those who had a double freeze–thaw cycle had a (–) biopsy rate of 93%.
- Single-cycle patients had a biochemical failure rate of 65%.
- Double-cycle patients had a biochemical failure rate of 44%.
- CONCLUSIONS:
  - Salvage cryotherapy is associated with high (–) biopsy rates and a low biochemical failure rate.
  - Double freeze–thaw cycles demonstrate statistically significantly higher efficacy than single cycles.

- Cryosurgery is an important option for salvage of post-radiation failure. However, longer follow-up is needed to determine the role of cryosurgery in the initial management of previously untreated prostate cancer.

Complications following cryosurgical ablation of the prostate

[Bahn DK, *Urology* **60**(2 Suppl 1): 3–11, 2002]
[Ellis D, *Urology* **60**(Suppl 2A): 34–39, 2002]
[Koppie TM, *J Urol* **162**: 427–432, 1999]
[Long JP, *J Urol* **159**(2): 477–484, 1998]

- Impotence.
  - Cryotherapy has the potential to compromise arterial flow to the penis and to damage the cavernosal nerves, both causative factors in erectile dysfunction.
  - Impotence rates vary in the range 40–93%.
  - The rate of regaining potency is in the range 5–13% for as long as 2 years post-treatment.
  - When compared to other modalities of locally controlling prostate cancer, cryotherapy is inferior with respect to preservation of potency.

- Incontinence.
  - Damage to the external urethral sphincter is a potential outcome of cryotherapy to the prostate.
  - Incontinence rates vary in the range 4–27% and depend greatly on the methods used to assess it. Nearly all studies have included incontinence as assessed by the physician, and not patient-reported data.

- Bahn et al. studied the largest patient population, and reported that 4.3% required 1 pad/day and that 11.6% required less than this.
- These rates are similar, if not lower, to those seen with other forms of local treatment for prostate cancer.

- Urethral tissue sloughing.
  - Freezing of the prostatic urethra can induce necrosis and sloughing in the area, and subsequently an increase in the risk of infection secondary to loss of the mucosal barrier. Tissue sloughing usually occurs 1–2 months post-treatment.
  - With the advent of urethral warming catheters, rates of sloughing were significantly reduced from 37% to 14%.
  - Urethral stricture is generally a result of tissue sloughing and subsequent scar formation.
  - Conservative treatment includes urinary drainage by continuous or intermittent catheterization, and antibiotics. More radical treatment is transurethral resection of the tissue.

- Rectourethral fistula.
  - Necrosis of the tissue posterior to the prostate gland, especially when associated with infection, can lead to fistula formation.
  - Rates are low (0–3%) in the larger retrospective studies.
  - Rates seem to have decreased since the use of argon gas instead of liquid nitrogen for cooling.
  - Formal repair of a fistula that does not respond to catheter drainage is postponed for 4–6 months post-treatment.

18

Adjuvant androgen suppression for locally advanced prostate cancer

Adjuvant androgen deprivation

- Radiation Therapy Oncology Group (RTOG) 85-31: indefinite androgen suppression adjuvant to radiation therapy (RT) in unfavorable prognosis prostate carcinoma (T_3 and/or node positive (N (+))) – long-term results.
  [Pilepich M, *Int J Radiat Oncol Biol Phys* **61**(5): 1285–1290, 2005]
  - 945 ♂: T_1–T_2 and N (+); or T_3 and N (±).
  - Staged clinically, or pathologically after prostatectomy.
  - Exclusions: bulky tumors (> 25 cm³) were excluded and placed on the parallel study (RTOG 86-10) for neoadjuvant hormone therapy.
  - *Unless* had N (+) *outside* the pelvis (common iliac or para-aortic), then placed on RTOG 85-31 for long-term adjuvant androgen deprivation (AD) regardless of whether had bulky disease.
  - Lymph node assessment mandatory (computerized tomography, lymphangiography, lymphadenectomy)
  - Group I: RT + goserelin (with AD starting during the last week of RT and continuing indefinitely or until disease progression).
  - Group II: RT + observation (with AD initiated at time of relapse).
  - RT: 44–50 Gy to whole pelvis, followed by a boost to the prostate for a total of 65–70 Gy, or to the prostatic bed for a total of 60–65 Gy after prostatectomy.
  - AD: Goserelin 3.6 mg s.c. q monthly.
  - RESULTS:
    See next page.

Endpoint	% at 10 years		
	Group I	Group II	p
Local failure	23	38	< 0.0001
Distant metastases	24	39	< 0.0001
NED survival	37	23	< 0.0001
bNED (PSA < 1.5 ng/ml)	31	9	< 0.0001
Absolute survival	**49**	**39**	0.002
Cause-specific mortality	16	22	0.0052

NED, no evidence of disease; bNED, biochemical NED.

- Subset analysis: survival benefit preferential for those with a Gleason score of 8–10, but absent in those with a Gleason score of 2–6.

Endpoint	% at 10 years		
	Group I	Group II	p
Gleason score 2–6			
Absolute survival	57	51	0.24
Cause-specific mortality	7	12	0.14
Gleason score 8–10			
Absolute survival	**39**	**25**	0.0046
Cause-specific mortality	27	40	0.0039

- CONCLUSIONS:
  - In this unfavorable population, adjuvant AD resulted in significant improvements in every endpoint, including survival, for the entire population.
  - Specifically, in T_3 and/or N (+) *and* with a high Gleason score of 8–10, there is a 10% benefit in overall survival (OS) at 10 years, and thus long-term AD may be the standard of care.
  - However, with its cost and morbidity, AD may not be justified in those with a Gleason score of 2–6.

- European Organisation for Research and Treatment of Cancer (EORTC) 22863: RT with concurrent and adjuvant AD × 3 years for locally advanced prostate cancer.
  [Bolla M, *Lancet* **360**: 103–108, 2002]

- 401 ♂ with T_1–T_2 and World Health Organization grade 3, or T_3–T_4, ± N disease (89% were T_3–T_4).
- Group I: RT alone.
- Group II: RT + goserelin starting on day 1 and continuing for 3 years.
- RT: 50 Gy to the whole pelvis, with additional 20 Gy to the prostate and seminal vesicles.
- AD: cyproterone acetate p.o. t.i.d. × 1 month beginning 1 week before goserelin, and goserelin s.c. q 4 weeks × 3 years starting on day 1 of RT.
- RESULTS:

Endpoint	% at 5 years		
	Group I	Group II	p
Local failure	16.4	1.7	< 0.0001
Distant metastases	29.2	9.8	< 0.0001
DFS	40	74	< 0.0001
Biochemical DFS	45	76	0.0001
Overall survival	**62**	**78**	0.0002
Cause-specific survival	79	94	0.0001

DFS, disease-free survival.

- CONCLUSIONS:
  - AD improves every endpoint, even **OS (16% at 5 years)**, irrespective of histologic grade (no preference for Gleason score).
  - AD may provide a method to improve on the outcome of external RT alone, possibly by eliminating occult systemic disease and by having an additive effect on local control.

Neoadjuvant androgen deprivation for locally advanced prostate cancer

- RTOG 86–10: neoadjuvant and concurrent AD with RT vs RT alone in bulky, locally advanced prostate carcinoma.
  [Pilepich M, *Int J Radiat Oncol Biol Phys* **50**(5): 1243–1252, 2001]
  - 456 ♂ with 'bulky' (> 25 cm³) T_2–T_4 tumors ± pelvic lymph node (LN) (not outside pelvis).
- Group I: combined androgen blockade (CAB) (*both* goserelin and flutamide) 2 months before and 2 months during RT.
- Group II: RT alone.

- RT: 44–50 Gy to the whole pelvis (± lower para-aortics), and boost of 65–72 Gy to the prostate.
- AD: goserelin 3.6 mg s.c. q 4 weeks and flutamide 250 mg p.o. t.i.d.
- Purpose: ↓ tumor bulk, ↑ tumor cell kill, and improve outcomes.
- RESULTS:

Endpoint	% at 8 years		
	Group I	Group II	p
Local failure	30	12	0.016
Distant metastases	34	45	0.04
NED	33	21	0.004
bNED (PSA < 1.5 ng/ml)	16	3	< 0.0001
Survival	53	44	0.10
Cause-specific mortality	23	31	0.05

NED, no evidence of disease; bNED, biochemical NED.

- Only local failure, NED, and bNED had statistically significant benefit.
- Subset analysis: Gleason score 7–10, no significant benefit in any endpoints (except bNED).
- However, there was a preferential benefit in those with a Gleason score of 2–6 for all endpoints, including survival.

Endpoint	Preferential benefit		
	Group I	Group II	p
Local failure	21	46	0.005
Distant metastases	13	34	0.006
NED	50	32	0.004
bNED (PSA < 1.5 ng/ml)	30	–	< 0.0001
Survival	70	52	0.015
Cause-specific mortality	2	17	0.0002

NED, no evidence of disease; bNED, biochemical NED.

- It is postulated that the mode of interaction between AD and RT varies depending on the timing and duration of AD.
  - Neoadjuvant AD may significantly debulk the tumor (cytoreduction), and ↓ tumor volume correlates with ↑ probability of control with RT.

- Concurrent AD may both ↑ tumor cell death (apoptosis) and ↓ the rate of tumor cell repopulation.
- SUMMARY:
  - Neoadjuvant and concurrent AD in bulky tumors with a Gleason score of 2–6 results in significant improvements in all endpoints, and may be the standard of care.

Neoadjuvant versus adjuvant androgen deprivation

- RTOG 92-02: short-term (neoadjuvant and concurrent) AD with RT vs long-term (neoadjuvant, concurrent, and adjuvant) AD with RT for locally advanced prostate carcinoma.
  [Hanks GE, *J Clin Oncol* **21**(21): 3972–3978, 2003]
  - Based on RTOG 85-31 (indefinite adjuvant AD) and RTOG 86-10 (neoadjuvant and concurrent AD), this study attempts to define the optimum duration of AD.
  - Standard group (the RTOG 86-10 schedule) vs investigational group (adjuvant AD × 2 years).
  - 1,514 ♂ with T_{2c}–T_4 tumors ± LN, but with no nodes in the common iliac or higher.
  - Group I: short-term AD for 2 months prior to and 2 months during RT (STAD-RT).
  - Group II: same as group I, but also long-term adjuvant AD for 24 months after RT (LTAD-RT) for a total of 28 months.
  - RT: 44–50 Gy to the whole pelvis, followed by a boost to the prostate of 65–70 Gy.
  - Combined androgen blockade (CAB): flutamide 250 mg p.o. t.i.d. with goserelin 3.6 mg q month.
  - RESULTS:

Endpoint	% at 5 years		
	STAD-RT	LTAD-RT	p
Local progression	12.3	6.4	0.0001
Distant metastases	17.0	11.5	0.0035
Biochemical failure	55.5	28.0	< 0.0001
Disease-free survival	**28.1**	**46.4**	< 0.0001
Overall survival	78.5	80.0	0.73
Cause-specific survival	**91.2**	**94.6**	0.006

- LTAD-RT group:
  - Significant advantage in all endpoints except OS.
  - Significant advantage in disease-free survival and cause-specific survival.
    - $\downarrow$ number of prostate cancer deaths but an $\uparrow$ number of deaths from other causes.
- For those with a Gleason score of 8–10, a significant advantage is seen in every endpoint, including OS.

Endpoint	% at 5 years		
	STAD-RT	LTAD-RT	p
Local progression	18.3	9.1	0.13
Distant metastases	27.3	15.5	0.004
Biochemical failure	65.0	33.4	< 0.0001
Disease-free survival	19.1	41.9	< 0.0001
Overall survival	**70.7**	**81.0**	0.044
Cause-specific survival	82.0	93.4	0.0078

- CONCLUSIONS:
  - For the entire group, a significant OS difference has not yet been observed at 5 years.
  - The results support RTOG 85-31.
  - LTAD has an advantage over STAD for those with a Gleason score of 8–10.
  - However, subset analysis of those with a Gleason score of 8–10 was not part of this study's initial protocol design, and should be interpreted with caution.
  - Because EORTC 22863 showed a 16% survival advantage at 5 years for all Gleason scores, and RTOG 85-31 showed a 10% survival advantage at 10 years for Gleason scores 8–10, we may expect to see an OS advantage in RTOG 92-02 with longer follow-up.

- Quebec study: RT alone vs neoadjuvant CAB with RT vs neoadjuvant, concurrent, and adjuvant CAB with RT.
  [Laverdiere J, *Int J Radiat Oncol Biol Phys* **37**(2): 247–252, 1997]
  - 120 σ with clinical stage T_{2a}–T_3 disease, randomized.
  - Three-group study:
    - Group I: RT alone.
    - Group II: neoadjuvant CAB × 3 months prior to RT.

- – Group III: neoadjuvant CAB × 3 months prior to, during, and 6 months after RT.
- RT: 64 Gy at 2 Gy/fraction to the whole pelvis.
- CAB: leuprolide acetate 7.5 mg i.m. q 4 weeks and flutamide 250 mg p.o. t.i.d..
- Endpoint: (+) biopsy rate and PSA level at 12 and 24 months.
- RESULTS:

Endpoint	Group I	Group II	Group III	p
% of (+) biopsy				
12 months	62	30	4	0.00005
24 months	65	28	5	< 0.00001
Median PSA level (ng/ml)				
12 months	1.56	0.6	0.2	
24 months	1.20	0.65	0.5	

- CONCLUSIONS:
  - – CAB in conjunction with RT results in statistically significantly lower rates of (+) biopsies than RT alone.
  - – The best results are when CAB is given in a prolonged and concomitant way.
  - – It is unknown if the benefit derives from a single factor (either concurrent CAB or prolonged CAB), or if both factors are involved.
- LIMITATION OF THE STUDY:
  - – RT was given at only 64 Gy; dose escalation would likely have resulted in a better outcome for the RT alone group.

Clinically localized prostate cancer

- RTOG 9413: whole-pelvis RT vs prostate-only RT and neoadjuvant CAB vs adjuvant CAB in prostate cancer with no clinical evidence of nodal disease.
  [Roach M, *J Clin Oncol* 21(10): 1904–1911, 2003]
  - 1,323 ♂ with localized prostate cancer with an estimated LN risk of > 15% and a PSA level ≤ 100 ng/ml.
  - Required to have an estimated risk of LN involvement of > 15% based on the equation:
    LN = (2/3)PSA + [(Gleason score − 6) × 10].

- ♂ with stage T_{2c}–T_4 disease were also eligible if they had a Gleason score ≥ 6, even if the LN risk was not $> 15\%$.
- 2×2 factorial design.
  - Group I: whole-pelvis RT + neoadjuvant and concurrent CAB.
  - Group II: prostate-only RT + neoadjuvant and concurrent CAB.
  - Group III: whole-pelvis RT + adjuvant CAB.
  - Group IV: prostate-only RT + adjuvant CAB.
- RT for whole-pelvis groups: 50.4 Gy to whole pelvis with an additional 19.8 Gy to the prostate using cone-down.
- RT for prostate-only groups: 70.2 Gy to the prostate and seminal vesicles only.
- AD: flutamide 250 mg p.o. t.i.d. + either goserelin 3.6 mg s.c. or leuprolide 7.5 mg i.m. q month.
- PSA failure was not the American Society for Therapeutic Radiology and Oncology (ASTRO) definition (as this was not designed for patients receiving hormone therapy) but was defined as 2 consecutive and 'significant' (≥ 0.3 ng/ml if the PSA ≤ 1.5 ng/ml, or $\geq 20\%$ if PSA > 1.5 ng/ml) PSA rises separated by at least 1 month.
- RESULTS:

Endpoint	% at 4 years				
	Group I	Group II	Group III	Group IV	p
Progression -free survival	60	44	49	50	0.008
PSA failure	30	43	37	37	0.048

  - Subset analysis: statistically significant difference in progression-free survival for intermediate-risk patients (Gleason score 2–6 and PSA ≥ 30 ng/ml, or Gleason score 7–10 and PSA < 30 ng/ml), but no difference for lowest risk patients (Gleason score 2–6 and PSA < 30 ng/ml) or highest risk patients (Gleason score 7–10 and PSA ≥ 30 ng/ml).
- CONCLUSIONS:
  - Whole-pelvis RT + neoadjuvant and concurrent CAB is the best of the four groups for patients with risk of LN (+) of $> 15\%$, with the greatest benefit in intermediate-risk patients.
  - The benefit cannot only be attributed to having a whole-pelvis field (i.e. missing the prostate or seminal vesicles with the prostate-only RT field), as whole-pelvis RT + adjuvant CAB did no better than prostate-only RT + adjuvant CAB, indicating

that the larger field size is not of benefit without neoadjuvant and concurrent CAB.
   - At the time of this follow-up, it was too early to detect an OS benefit.

- Short-term (6 month) androgen suppression + 70 Gy three-dimensional conformal radiation therapy (3D-CRT) vs 70 Gy 3D-CRT alone for clinically localized, intermediate- to high-risk prostate cancer. [D'Amico A, JAMA **292**(7): 821–827, 2004]
  - 206 ♂ with T_{1b}–T_{2b} disease, and a PSA of 10–40 ng/ml or a Gleason score ≥ 7.
  - Group I: CAB $\times$ 2 months prior to, 2 months during, and 2 months after RT.
  - Group II: RT alone.
  - RT: 1.8 Gy for 45 Gy and then 2 Gy for 11 Gy for total of 70.35 Gy (67 Gy normalized to 95%) to the prostate only plus a 1.5-cm margin using 3D-CRT.
  - AD: Flutamide 250 mg p.o. t.i.d. + either leuprolide (7.5 mg i.m. q month or 22.5 mg q 3 months) or goserelin (3.6 mg s.c. q month or 10.8 mg s.c. q 3 months).
- RESULTS:

Endpoint	% at 5 years		
	Group I	Group II	p
Overall survival	88	78	0.04
Cause-specific mortality	0	5.8	0.02
Survival without salvage androgen-suppression therapy	82	57	0.002

- CONCLUSIONS:
  - Short-term androgen-suppression therapy (AST) conferred a survival benefit for clinically localized, but intermediate- to high-risk prostate cancer.
  - Questions remain:
    - Could survival have been increased further if a higher dose (78 Gy) was used or if pelvic LNs were irradiated?
    - Is AST even necessary in the setting of RT dose escalation?
    - Should the short-term AST be given prior to, concurrently with or adjuvantly with RT?
    - Is short-term AST sufficient, or is long-term AST needed? (This question is currently being addressed by RTOG 9408 and EORTC 22961.)

Current phase III trials

- RTOG 9408 – to evaluate AD for earlier stage disease.
    - Neoadjuvant and concurrent CAB (2 months prior to and during) with RT for locally confined prostate cancer (T_{1b}–T_{2b} and PSA ≤ 20 ng/ml).

- RTOG 9910 – to evaluate a longer duration of neoadjuvant therapy.
    - Neoadjuvant CAB $\times$ 2 months before vs $\times$ 7 months before, and during RT for stage T_{1b}–T_4, Gleason score 2–6, and PSA > 10 ng/ml; or T_{1b}–T_4, Gleason score 7, and PSA 20 ng/ml; or T_{1b}–T_{1c}, Gleason score 8–10, and PSA < 20 ng/ml.

- RTOG 9902 – to evaluate the addition of chemotherapy to AD for unfavorable disease.
    - Neoadjuvant, concurrent, and adjuvant AD $\times$ 2 years $\pm$ chemotherapy for high-risk prostate cancer (Gleason score ≥ 7 and PSA 20–100 ng/ml; or T_2–T_3, Gleason score 8, and PSA ≤ 100 ng/ml).

- EORTC 22961 – to compare short-term vs long-term adjuvant AD.
    - CAB $\times$ 6 months during and after RT $\pm$ luteinizing hormone releasing hormone (LHRH) $\times$ 30 months in $T_{1c-2b}N_1$ or $T_{1c-4}N_{0-2}$.

- EORTC 22991 – AD for intermediate-risk disease.
    - RT alone vs RT + LHRH $\times$ 6 months during and after RT + non-steroidal antiandrogen (Casodex) $\times$ 1 month for stage T_{1b}–T_{1c} and PSA > 10 ng/ml and/or Gleason score ≥ 7, or T_{2a}.

Summary of the trials

- Although the use of *adjuvant* therapy may improve local control, the primary purpose is to the extend the duration of freedom from relapse and improve disease-specific survival by preventing growth of clinically occult *metastases*.

- Long-term data from RTOG 85-31 show a survival benefit with indefinite adjuvant AD for the *entire* population of unfavorable (T_3 or N (+)) patients, although it is preferential for high Gleason scores of 7–10.

- EORTC 22863 shows a survival benefit with concurrent and adjuvant CAB $\times$ 3 years for the entire group of locally advanced disease, regardless of histologic grade.

- The rationale for *neoadjuvant* therapy is for *cytoreduction*, because a smaller tumor volume correlates with better local control with RT.

- The rationale for *concurrent* therapy is *enhanced apoptosis* and $\downarrow$ *repopulation*.

- RTOG 86-10 shows a significant OS benefit with neoadjuvant and concurrent CAB for 'bulky' T_2–T_4 tumors, but only with low Gleason scores of 2–6 (not seen for Gleason scores 7–10).

- RTOG 92-02 shows that long-term (neoadjuvant, concurrent, and adjuvant) AD was better than short-term (neoadjuvant and adjuvant) AD, especially in those with a high Gleason score of 8–10 (in agreement with RTOG 85–31).

- RTOG 94-13 shows that neoadjuvant and concurrent AD + whole-pelvis radiation therapy(WPRT) was better than adjuvant AD + WPRT in those with clinically localized disease but a (+) LN risk of > 15%.

- D'Amico's study showed a survival benefit with short-term (2 months prior to, 2 months during, and 2 months after) AD with 3D-CRT for early localized disease.

19

Prostate cancer recurrence

Biochemical recurrence

[Kuban DA, J Urol 173(6): 1871–1878, 2005]
[Swindle PW, Urol Clin North Am 30: 377–401, 2003]
[Vicini FA, J Urol 173: 1456–1462, 2005]

- American Society for Therapeutic Radiology and Oncology (ASTRO)/ Radiation Therapy Oncology Group (RTOG) 2005 Consensus Statement.
  [Roade M, Int J Radiat Oncol Biol Phys 65(4): 965–974, 2006]
  - Rise of prostate-specific antigen (PSA) ≥ 2 ng/ml above the nadir PSA (nPSA) after external beam radiation therapy (EBRT) with or without hormone therapy.
  - Date of failure is determined 'at call' (not backdated).
  - To avoid the artifacts resulting from short follow-up, the reported date of control should be listed as 2 years short of the median follow-up.
    - For example, if the median follow-up is 5 years, control rates at 3 years should be cited.
    - Retaining a strict version of the ASTRO definition would allow comparisons with a large existing body of literature.

- The ASTRO 1996 definition of biochemical failure/recurrence is:
  - Not equivalent to clinical failure.
  - Biochemical failure is not justification per se to initiate additional treatment.

- However, it is an appropriate early endpoint for clinical trials.
- PSA determinations should be obtained at 3- or 4-month intervals during the first 2 years after the completion of radiation therapy and every 6 months thereafter.
  - Three consecutive PSA ↑ represent a reasonable definition of biochemical failure after radiation therapy.
  - For clinical trials the date of failure should be the midpoint between the post-radiation nPSA and the first of the three consecutive increases.
- To date no definition of PSA failure has been shown to be a surrogate for clinical progression or survival.
- The nPSA is a strong prognostic factor, but no absolute level is a valid cut-off point for separating successful and unsuccessful therapy.

- Critique of the 1996 ASTRO definition.
  1. Does not define what the magnitude of rise should reach to be considered 'significant'.
  2. Does not define which nPSA to use: lowest ever (*absolute nPSA*) vs nPSA just antecedent to the rise (*current nPSA*).
  3. Back-dates biochemical failure to a time midway between the nPSA and the first rise.
  4. Does not take into account 'bumps'.
  5. Greater specificity and sensitivity of other definitions (see below).
  6. Meaning is unclear after brachytherapy. No extrapolation is possible to cover post-radical prostatectomy failure.

- Alternative definitions of biochemical recurrence exist.
  - Vancouver Rules.
    [Pickles T, *Int J Radiat Oncol Biol Phys* **43**(3): 699–700, 1999]
    - Either of two situations:
      - Failure to achieve an nPSA of ≤ 4 ng/ml 1 year post-radiation therapy, <u>OR</u>
      - Two criteria have to be fulfilled: (i) ≥ 2 rises ≥ 1 month apart ABOVE the 'reference nadir' (nPSA not followed by a subsequent fall) <u>AND</u> (ii) PSA ≥ 1.5 ng/ml.

- [Horwitz EM, *J Urol* **173**: 797–802, 2002]
  - Assessed 102 definitions of biochemical recurrence for the largest data set available to date (4,839 patients).
  - Using clinical failure (+ biopsy, + digital rectal examination, or radiographic evidence) as the gold standard, three definitions were found to be superior to the ASTRO definition.

Definition	Distant + local		Distant only	
	Sens. (%)	Spec. (%)	Sens. (%)	Spec. (%)
ASTRO 1996 definition	60	72	55	68
> 'Current nadir + 3'	66	77	76	72
> 'Absolute nadir + 2' (Houston definition)	64	74	72	70
Two consecutive rises (each ≥ 0.5 ng/ml)	67	78	79	72

Sens., sensitivity; spec., specificity.

- Biochemical recurrence is usually the first evidence of disease recurrence, and almost invariably occurs in isolation without any objective findings.

- It has been demonstrated that the overall survival rate of patients at 10 years was equal in patients with and without biochemical recurrence. [Jhaveri FM, *Urology* **54**: 884–890, 1999]

Biochemical recurrence after radiation therapy

- With radiation the secretory function of the prostate, although markedly reduced, is usually not totally ablated.

- Radiation therapy produces a general downward trend in PSA, typically over 1.5–3 years, but not without substantial individual variation and fluctuation secondary to what can be a benign etiology instead of tumor.

- Predictors of biochemical recurrence.
  - Preoperative PSA level.
  - Pathologic T stage.
  - Gleason score (biopsy and prostatectomy).
  - Margin status.
  - Lymph node (LN) involvement.
  - Seminal vesicle involvement.
  - Perineural invasion.
  - Tumor volume.
  - Treatment factors include the modality of radiotherapy used (i.e. conventional, three-dimensional conformal, or intensity-modulated conformal).

- Prognostic factors for the development of metastatic disease.
  - Time to biochemical progression: early PSA relapse < 12 months.
  - Gleason score.
  - PSA doubling time: rapid post-irradiation PSA doubling time < 12 months.

Biochemical recurrence after surgery

[Scattoni V, *BJU Int* **93**: 680–688, 2004]

- The definition of 'disease-free' after surgery is more straightforward, as the entire PSA-producing organ has been removed.

- Following surgery, the PSA should fall to undetectable levels within 4 weeks.
  - The half-life of PSA is 3.15 days.

- Although varying levels of PSA are used to define failure after surgery, a rising PSA should alert one to possible failure.

- Predictors of freedom from biochemical recurrence after radical retropubic prostatectomy.
  - Lower clinical stage.
  - Gleason score at biopsy.
  - PSA level.
  - No extracapsular extension.
  - (–) surgical margins.
  - Lower Gleason scores.

Treatment of biochemical recurrence

[Dreicer R, *Cancer Treat Rev* **28**: 189–194, 2002]

- There is no 'standard of care' for the management of patients with biochemical failure.

- Immediate vs deferred androgen suppression remains controversial.

- Some infer that biochemical recurrence is a presumption of systemic failure.

- Several studies have attempted to guide the timing of hormone therapy.

- VACURG I (Veterans Administration Cooperative Urological Research Group).
  [Blackard CE, *Urology* **1**(6): 553–560, 1973]

- In one group 262 patients with locally advanced ($T_{3-4}M_0$) disease were assigned to placebo and 266 to orchiectomy.
- In another group 223 patients with metastatic disease were assigned to placebo, and 203 patients were assigned to orchiectomy.
- RESULTS:
  - At 9-year follow-up there was no difference in disease-specific or overall survival, suggesting a lack of benefit from early hormone therapy.

- VACURG II.
  [Byar DP, *Cancer* **32**: 1126–1130, 1973]
  - Randomized > 1,500 patients with locally advanced and metastatic disease into four groups: placebo, and diethylstilbestrol (DES) 0.2, 1 and 5 mg/day.
  - RESULTS:
    - There was a suggestion that the 1 mg dose of DES provided a survival advantage, but this is questionable due to the fact that the 5 mg dose was associated with an excess of cardiovascular deaths, and the placebo and 0.2 mg DES groups had protocol issues.

- European Organisation for Research and Treatment of Cancer (EORTC) 22863.
  [Bolla M, *N Engl J Med* **337**: 295–300, 1997]
  - Randomized 401 patients with either high-grade $T_{1-2}N_0$ or T_3/T_4 any grade patients to radiotherapy alone or radiotherapy + androgen ablation (goserelin) for 3 years.
  - RESULTS:
    - At 5 years the survival of patients receiving radiotherapy + androgen ablation was 79%, vs 62% for radiotherapy alone.

- Eastern Cooperative Oncology Group (ECOG) 3886/Southwest Oncology Group (SWOG) 8793.
  [Messing EM, *N Engl J Med* **341**: 1781–1789, 1999]
  - Randomized, prospective study of immediate hormone therapy (either with goserelin monthly or orchiectomy) vs observation in ♂ undergoing radical prostatectomy with evidence of (+) LNs.
  - 98 patients total.
  - Median follow-up → 7.1 years.
  - RESULTS:
    - 7/47 ♂ who received immediate antiandrogen therapy had died compared with 18/51 in the observation group ($p = 0.02$).
  - LIMITATIONS OF THE STUDY:

- Small sample size, lack of central pathologic review, and relatively low cancer-specific survival rate in the control group.

- Medical Research Council (MRC).
  [MRC Prostate Cancer Working Party Investigators Group, *Br J Urol* 79: 235–246, 1997]
  - Randomized trial of immediate vs deferred therapy for advanced prostate cancer.
  - 934 evaluable patients.
  - RESULTS:
    - Disease-specific survival is statistically significant, but overall survival for patients with locally advanced disease receiving immediate therapy is not significantly different from those in the delayed group.

- Androgen deprivation has problems.
  - Loss of libido.
  - Loss of potency.
  - Hot flashes.
  - Fatigue.
  - Anemia.
  - Loss of muscle mass.
  - Weight gain.
  - Depression.
  - Osteoporosis.
  - ↓ quality of life.

- Hormone therapy is a temporizing measure.

- Predictive factors for recurrence and prognostic factors should guide the initiation of immediate vs delayed hormone therapy in individual patients.

Local recurrence

[Scattoni V, *BJU Int* **93**: 680–688, 2004]

- Local recurrence after radical retropubic prostatectomy refers to the documentation of disease in the prostatic fossa, either by biopsy or digital rectal examination, whereas local recurrence post-radiation therapy is suggested by a (+) prostate biopsy 1–2 years after therapy.

- In patients with biochemical failure post-radiation therapy, it is difficult to identify reliably those with solely 'local' vs those with 'distant' failure.

- The diagnosis of local failure is often *inferred or presumed* based on knowledge of clinical predictors.

Clinical predictors of local vs distant failure

- The lower the nodic PSA (nPSA), the more likely the failure is local than distant.
  - The median nPSA values for local vs distant failure were 1.1 ng/ml vs 2.2 ng/ml, respectively.
  [Crook J, *Int J Radiat Oncol Biol Phys* **48**: 355–367, 2002]

- The longer the PSA doubling time, the greater the probability of local vs distant failure.

  PSA doubling time = 0.693(Duration between measurements)/
  $\qquad$ (ln 2nd PSA – ln 1st PSA).

  - A PSA doubling time ≤ 6 months is more suggestive of local failure, whereas a PSA doubling time > 6 months is more suggestive of distant failure.
  [Sartor C, *Int J Radiat Oncol Biol Phys* **38**: 941–947, 1997]

- On multivariate analysis of 1,540 patients, all of whom were treated with EBRT for biochemical failure after radical retropubic prostatectomy (RRP), the following variables led to the development of a nomogram to identify those who would benefit from salvage EBRT (i.e. those in whom recurrence is more likely to be local).
  1. PSA level after RRP: if ≤ 0.5 ng/ml, more likely to benefit.
  2. PSA doubling time: if ≤ 10 months, more likely to benefit.
  3. Gleason score on prostatectomy specimen: if ≥ 8, more likely to benefit.
  4. LN metastases.

Diagnostic studies before treatment of local failure or 'inferred/presumed' local failure: bone scan and CT of the pelvis (Table 19.1)

- The rate of (+) biopsy after radiotherapy varies from 25% to 32% (except in one study of 27 patients where 93% had a (+) biopsy), depending on the study and length of study (Table 19.2).
  [Touma NJ, *J Urol* **173**(2): 373–379, 2005]

- Following radiotherapy three parameters have been consistently identified as predictors of local failure: the nPSA, time to the nadir, and the PSA doubling time.

- Using these three factors, patients can be stratified into three distinct risk groups of radiation therapy failure.
  - The 5-year PSA relapse-free rate is 75–85% in the low-risk group, 58–65% in the intermediate group, and 35–38% in the high-risk group.

Table 19.1 Utility of investigations for the identification of the site of disease recurrence

Investigation	Local recurrence	Metastatic disease
Transrectal ultrasound (TRUS) and biopsy	Minimal role post-RRP. Used to document persistent disease if salvage RRP is considered following failed radiotherapy	NA
Compterized tomography (CT)	Minimal utility for the early identification of local recurrence post-RRP	Useful for identification of advanced nodal, visceral, or bony disease
Bone scan	NA	Minimal role for the investigation of early biochemical recurrence. Indicated if there is a rapid change in PSA level or the PSA level is > 10–20 ng/ml
Magnetic resonance imaging (MRI)	Encouraging early results. Await further validation	Encouraging results for early detection of bony metastases. Await further validation
ProstaScint	Should be used only in a protocol setting. Await further validation	Should be used only in protocol setting. Await further validation
Positron emission tomography (PET)	Minimal role	Minimal role

NA, not available; PSA, prostate-specific antigen; RRP, radical retropubic prostatectomy.

Table 19.2 Positive biopsy rates after radiotherapy

Study	No. of patients	Post-radiotherapy biopsy time	(+) Biopsy (%)
Scardino & Wheeler	140	6–36 months	32
Kabalin et al	27	5.2 years	93
Borghede et al	131	18 months	25
Crook et al	498	Median 13–55 months	27
Zelefsky et al	252	> 2.5 years	27
Pollack et al	168	2 years	30

[From: Touma NJ, *J Urol* **173**(2): 373–379, 2005]

Treatment modalities for local recurrence after radiation therapy

- Treatment should be individualized to the patient.

- Local failure was found to be a strong predictor of distant metastasis. [Coen JJ, *J Clin Oncol* **20**: 3199–3205, 2002]

- Options for treatment after radiation therapy.
  1. Hormone manipulation (discussed under biochemical recurrence, see page 204).
  2. Salvage surgery.
  3. Salvage brachytherapy.
  4. Salvage cryotherapy.

Salvage radical prostatectomy (Table 19.3)

- Operating in an irradiated field has proved to be a challenge, resulting in significant complications.

- Patient selection is important for outcome, and the ideal patient has:
  - A life expectancy of at least 10 years.
  - A lack of severe medical comorbidities.
  - High motivation and acceptance of ↑ surgical morbidity.
  - A pre-radiation PSA < 10 ng/ml.
  - A preoperative PSA < 10 ng/ml.
  - A pre-radiation localized clinical stage and a preoperative localized clinical stage.

- There is still a question about whether preoperative clinical stage (extraprostatic involvement) determines disease-free survival rates.

- One study suggested that preoperative patients with a localized clinical stage preoperatively show a trend toward better disease-free survival rates than those with clinically evident extraprostatic involvement ($p = 0.09$).
[Gheiler E, *Urology* **51**: 789–795, 1998]

- In contrast, another study found that preoperative clinical stage was not a predictor of outcome.
  - Moreover, this study did not find an impact of biopsy Gleason score on pathological stage.

- There is no consensus regarding pelvic LN dissection during salvage prostatectomy, but most investigators generally recommend pelvic lymphadenectomy.

Table 19.3	Results of salvage radical prostatectomy				
Study	No. of patients	Follow-up (months)	Organ-confined disease (%)	SVI (%)	Biochemical NED (%)
Amling et al	108	NA	39	N/A	43*
Gheiler et al[†]	40	36.1	39.5	28.9	47
Garzotto & Wajsman[†]	29	63.6	28	NA	69
Rogers et al	40	39.3	20	49	47
Pontes et al[†]	43	12–120	30	58.2	25.6
Ahlering et al[†]	34	53.5	35	NA	64.7
Stein et al[†]	13	NA	38.5	46.2	NA
Link & Freiha	14	18	30.8	54	46
Neerhut et al	16	20	25	62.5	86[‡]

SVI, seminal vesicle involvement.
*Actuarial 10-year biochemical no evidence of disease (NED).
[†] Including cystoprostatectomy.
[‡] Distant metastasis survival, no PSA follow-up.

- Pathological findings at salvage prostatectomy are predictors of post-operative outcome.
  - There is still a debate about whether there is a survival advantage of lower Gleason scores.
  - DNA ploidy status of the prostatectomy specimen was found to be an independent predictor of outcome in the Mayo Clinic data.
  - Patients with DNA diploid tumors attained a better cancer-specific survival rate than did those with aneuploid tumors. Patients with tetraploid tumors had an intermediate survival rate.

- Salvage radical prostatectomy is more technically challenging than primary radical prostatectomy due to radiation-induced vasculitis, fibrosis, and tissue plane obliteration, which can lead to rectal injuries (0–9%), stricture (0–20%), and urinary incontinence (≤ 80%).

Salvage cryoablation of the prostate

- A problem of post-cryosurgery follow-up is that no clear definition of failure has been agreed on, and thus biochemical no evidence of disease (NED) rates vary widely according to the definition of failure used.

- It has been demonstrated that complete ablation of the prostate is not usually attained.

- Preoperative PSA levels, biopsy Gleason scores, and clinical stage appear to correlate with biochemical outcome.

- A pre-cryotherapy PSA < 10 ng/ml and lower grade Gleason score (≤ 8) are predictors of a sustained biochemical response.
  [Izawa J, *J Clin Oncol* **20**: 2664–2671, 2002]

- Pre-radiotherapy clinical stage < T_3 is associated with superior biochemical-relapse-free rates.

- Patients who received hormone therapy in addition to radiotherapy prior to cryosurgery appear to have a poorer outcome than those receiving radiotherapy alone.
  [Pisters L, *J Clin Oncol* **17**: 2514–2520, 1999]

- Intraoperative and postoperative parameters have been identified as having an impact on outcome.
  - Double freeze–thaw cycles are superior to a single freeze–thaw cycle for achieving biochemical NED and (–) biopsies.
  - The number of cryoprobes used is also a determinant of more complete glandular ablation: up to 8 cryoprobes in selected cases instead of the more commonly used 5 probes.

- While cryosurgery is relatively effective for local cancer control, it has limited capacity for complete prostate cryoablation. Therefore, legitimate concern exists regarding the potential for future tumor recurrence.

Salvage brachytherapy

- Brachytherapy has been reported as another potential salvage option when external radiation fails.

- The 5-year biochemical NED rate was 34% using two consecutive PSA increases above the nadir as the definition of failure.

- It is NOT as commonly used as other salvage options due to the limited radiation that can be given with the implants.

Treatment modalities for local recurrence after surgery

[Scattoni V, *BJU Int* **93**: 680–688, 2004]

- Key to determining which therapy to use is to try to determine whether the failure is local or metastatic (Table 19.4).

- Predictors of local recurrence:
  - Gleason score < 7.
  - No seminal vesicle invasion.
  - (–) pelvic LNs.
  - PSA detectable > 1 year after radical prostatectomy.
  - PSA velocity < 0.75 ng/ml per year.
  - PSA doubling time ≥ 6 months.

- Predictors of distant metastases:
  - Gleason score ≥ 7.
  - Seminal vesicle invasion.
  - (+) pelvic LNs.
  - PSA detectable < 1 year after radical prostatectomy.
  - PSA velocity > 0.75 ng/ml per year.
  - PSA doubling time ≥ 6 months.

- Patients with a Gleason score > 8, (+) seminal vesicles, or LN metastases have a 95%, 86%, and 100% likelihood of developing metastatic disease, respectively.
  [Han M, *Urol Clin North Am* **28**: 555–565, 2001]
  [Han M, *J Urol* **169**: 517–523, 2003]

Table 19.4 Variables associated with recurrence

Variable	Local recurrence	Distant metastases ± local recurrence
No. of patients	41 (34%)	88 (66%)
Gleason score:		
2–4	0	0
5–6	55%	45%
7	39%	61%
8–10	11%	89%
Pathological stage:		
organ confined	40%	60%
capsular penetration	54%	46%
Negative margins:		
capsular penetration	48%	52%
Positive surgical margins:		
seminal-vesicle involvement	16%	84%
LN metastases	7%	93%
Timing of PSA recurrence		
In 1 year	7%	93%
Within 1–2 years	10%	90%
After year 2	61%	39%
After year 3	74%	26%

Reproduced with kind permission of AW Partin.
[Partin AW, *Urology* **43**: 649–659, 1994]

- Conversely, biochemical relapse is more likely due to local failure alone if there are multiple (+) surgical margins, extensive extra-capsular disease, Gleason score ≤ 7, and no nodal or seminal-vesicle involvement.
  [Anscher MS, *Int J Radiat Oncol Biol Phys* **21**: 941–947, 1991]
  [Nudell DM, *Urology* **54**: 1049–1057, 1999]
  [Kupelian P, *Urology* **48**: 249–260, 1996]

- Diagnostic aids for post-radical prostatectomy local failure.
  1. Digital rectal examination.

- Not useful if PSA is undetectable.
  [Obek C, J Urol **162**: 762–764, 1999]
- Outcome is likely to improve if local recurrence is identified before disease is palpable.
2. Urethrovesicle anastomosis biopsy.
   - (+) in 41–60% of post-radical prostatectomy biochemical failure.
   - (+) biopsy does not predict outcome of salvage radiation therapy.
     [Koppie TM, J Urol **166**: 111–115, 2001]
   - Hence it is not routinely obtained for diagnosis of local failure.
3. Skeletal scintigraphy and pelvic computerized tomography (CT).
   - Average PSA values for a (+) bone scan and CT scan are 61.3 ng/ml and 27 ng/ml, respectively.
     [Kane CJ, Urology **61**: 607–611, 2003]
   - [^{111}In]Capromab pentitide (ProstaScint).
   - Monoclonal murine antibody against prostate-specific membrane antigen is expressed by normal prostatic epithelium, but to a much higher extent by prostate cancer cells.
   - Mean PSA for a (+) scan: 8.9 ng/ml.
     [Sodee DB, Clin Nuclear Med **21**: 759–767, 1996]
   - Hinckle 1998:

	Recurrence found using:	
	Indium-111 study	Pelvic CT or MRI
Sensitivity for LNs	75%	20%
Specificity	85%	68%
Positive predictive value	80%	30%

   - 255 patients with clinically localized disease were treated definitively with radical prostatectomy and followed by PSA determination and [^{111}In]Capromab.
     [Raj GV, Cancer **94**(4): 987–996, 2002]
     - RESULTS:
       - 72% overall had (+) scans, 31% were (+) only in the prostatic fossa.
       - In any group (stratified by PSA) about 1/3 of scans were (+) for distant sites.
       - The proportion of scans that were (+) only in the prostatic fossa for each PSA-defined group ranged from 25.3% (for PSA < 0.5 ng/ml) to 30.6% (for PSA ≤ 4 ng/ml).

- CONCLUSIONS:
  - Further studies are needed to define better the role of this diagnostic tool.
4. Positron emission tomography (PET).
   - Of limited value with [^{18}F]fluoro-2-deoxyglucose ([^{18}F]FDG) but the use of [^{11}C]choline may improve the utility of PET.

- Options of treatment of post-radical prostatectomy local failure.
  1. External beam radiotherapy (EBRT).
  2. Other, less frequently used options:
     - High-intensity focused ultrasound (HIFU): this is still experimental.
     - Brachytherapy: the role for this is unclear.

- Patient selection is an important component of choosing therapy.

- The timing and dose of radiotherapy also impacts on PSA-free survival.

- The ASTRO Consensus Panel recommended salvage EBRT be given when the PSA level is < 1.5 ng/ml.
  - The PSA cut-off to trigger salvage EBRT is variable.
  - Initiating salvage radiotherapy with a PSA of 1.0 ng/ml is likely to confer the best chance of biochemical survival.

- The dose of radiation is important in terms of biochemical-disease-free survival after salvage therapy.
  - Several studies have shown that a dose of > 64.8 Gy is a significant prognostic factor for biochemical-recurrence-free survival.

- No definitive studies are available to clarify the volume that should be irradiated (i.e. the prostatic fossa only or the whole pelvis).

- [Kim BS, *Clin Prostate Cancer* **3**(2): 93–97, 2004]
  A retrospective study of 42 patients at the University of Michigan with post-radical prostatectomy biochemical failure who received salvage EBRT (either through 'extended fields' that encompassed the whole pelvis followed by reduced fields to the prostatic fossa alone, or through 'limited' fields to the prostatic fossa only).
  - The doses given in both patient groups were similar.
  - No statistically significant differences were noted in any of the endpoints assessing outcome.

20

Metastatic prostate cancer

Management of bone metastases

[Carlin BI, *Cancer* **88**: 2989–2994, 2000]
[Pinski J, *Eur J Cancer* **41**: 932–940, 2005]

- Bone metastases are a common complication of prostate cancer.
  - 85% of ♂ who die from prostate cancer have bone metastases.

- The most common sequelae of bone metastases are:
  - Bone pain, debility, pathological fractures, and cord compression.

- Hypercalcemia of malignancy is rarely seen in prostate cancer.

- However, prostate bone lesions are typically sclerotic due to stimu-lation of osteoblasts.
  - Nevertheless, bone resorption is also enhanced, and the net effect is bone loss.

- Technetium-99m bone scans are generally used to detect bone metastases.
  [Rosenthal D, *Cancer* **80**: 1595–1607, 1997]
  - Although they are sensitive for metastases, they are not specific.
  - ↑ tracer uptake can occur at sites of degenerative changes, trauma, and infection.

- Magnetic resonance imaging (MRI) of the spine can detect sites of disease which are not apparent on a bone scan.
  - However, MRI is associated with a high false-positive rate and must be interpreted cautiously.

Management of painful bone metastases

[Payne R, *Cancer* **80**: 1608–1613, 1997]

- Clinical characteristics.
  - Bone pain is the commonest result of bone metastases.
  - Pain results from pending or pathological fractures, ↑ intraosseous pressure, and periosteal elevation.
  - Bone pain is often described by patients as a dull ache which is localized to a specific bone.
    - It is often more intense at night.
  - Bone pain may be aggravated by movement (often termed 'incident pain'), weight bearing, or both.
    - Incident pain is characteristic of bone metastases, and is defined as pain accentuation that is out of keeping with the nature of the associated movement.
    - Incident pain predicts for a poor outcome for symptom control. [Portenoy R, *Pain* **41**: 273–281, 1990]
- Opioid analgesics and non-steroidal anti-inflammatory drugs (NSAIDs) are very effective in ameliorating most instances of bone pain.

External beam radiotherapy

[Chow E, *World J Urol* **21**: 229–242, 2003]
[Sze W, *Clin Oncol* **15**: 345–352, 2003]

- External beam radiation therapy (EBRT) remains the mainstay of treating symptomatic bone metastases. However, there is no clear consensus on the optimum dose fractionation.

- Multifractionated radiation therapy generally results in more complete and longer durable pain relief than single fractions. [Ratanatharathorn V, *Int J Radiat Oncol Biol Phys* **44**: 1–18, 1999]

- Meta-analysis of dose fractionation radiation therapy for palliation of painful bone metastases. [Wu J, *Int J Radiat Oncol Biol Phys* **55**: 594–605, 2003]
  - There was no difference in complete or overall pain relief between single and multi-fraction palliative radiation therapy.

- European oncologists have largely adopted a single treatment of 8 Gy as standard practice; whereas, North American oncologists more typically prescribe multiple fractions to a total dose of 20–30 Gy.

Hemibody radiation

- Radiation Therapy Oncology Group (RTOG) 8206.
  [Poulter C, *Int J Radiat Oncol Biol Phys* **23**: 207–214, 1992]
  - 499 patients were randomized to receive hemibody radiation (HBI) (a single 8 Gy fraction) or no further treatment following standard local field radiation therapy.
  - RESULTS:
    - Improvement was seen in time to progression at 1 year with HBI (35% vs 46%, $p = 0.032$).
    - Using the multiple hazards model, the extent of metastases was the most significant factor influencing the time to progression; the site of the primary tumor was not.
    - Time to new disease within the hemibody field was delayed with HBI (12.6 vs 6.3 months).
    - Grade 3 or 4 hematological toxicity was higher in the HBI group (7.6% vs 0.5%, $p = 0.004$).
  - LIMITATIONS OF THE STUDY:
    - All primary tumor sites were included and were not controlled for in the study, although variable radiosensitivity was expected.
    - Effects of other interventions were not controlled.
    - Time to progression was dependent on the frequency of evaluations.
  - CONCLUSIONS:
    - HBI may have a limited role in preventing symptomatic progression in some tumor sites.
    - Significant hematological toxicity is anticipated.
    - HBI is not generally recommended in addition to local radiation therapy to painful sites.

Radionuclides

[McEwan A, *Semin Radiat Oncol* **10**: 103–114, 2000]

- Patients often have multiple sites of bone metastases, some of which are symptomatic, and they therefore may require several courses of radiation therapy to different painful sites.

- Radionuclides, such as strontium-89 or sumarium-153, have an affinity to bone and concentrate in areas of ↑ bone tumor, such as sites of osteoblastic metastases.

- Contraindications to radiopharmaceuticals.
  - Extensive soft tissue metastases.

- Platelet count < 60,000/ml.
- White blood count < 2500/ml.
- Disseminated intravascular coagulation.
- Projected survival < 2 months.
- HBI within the previous 2 months.
- Myelosuppressive chemotherapy within 1 month.
- Impending or established pathological fracture or spinal cord compression.

- Strontium-89 (^{89}Str).
  - Injectable radionuclide.
  - Emits β-particles; half-life 50.5 days.
  - Dose: 4 mCi.
  - Pain relief occurs within 3 months in 50–70% of patients.
  - Duration of pain relief: 20–30 weeks.

- Strontium-89 vs HBI vs EBRT.
  [Quilty P, *Radiother Oncol* **31**: 33, 1994]
  - 284 ♂ with prostate cancer and painful bone metastasis were randomized to three groups.
    - Group I: strontium-89.
    - Group II: HBI.
    - Group III: EBRT.
  - Pain sites were assessed at 4, 8, and 12 weeks post-therapy.
  - RESULTS:
    - All treatments provided pain relief.
    - At 3 months pain relief was sustained.
      - HBI → 63.6%.
      - EBRT → 61%.
      - Strontium-89 → 66%.
    - Fewer patients reported new sites of pain with strontium-89 than with EBRT.
    - Radiotherapy to new sites was required in 12 patients after EBRT vs 2 patients after strontium-89.
    - Platelet and leukocyte ↓ occurred in ~ 30–40% of patients, but sequelae were rare.

- Samarium-153 (^{153}Sm) bound to ethylenediamine-tetra(methylene phosphonic acid) (EDTMP).
  - Radioactive samarium-153 bound to the tetraphosphonate chelator EDTMP.
  - Injectable.
  - Emits β-particles; half-life 46 hours.

- – Similar uptake in bone to technetium-99 (^{99}Tc).
- – Recommended dose: 1.0 mCi/kg.

- Randomized, placebo-controlled study of samarium-153.
  [Serafini A, *J Clin Oncol* **16**: 1574–1581, 1998]
  - 118 patients with painful bone metastases (68% had prostate cancer) randomized to samarium-153 0.5 or 1 mCi/kg or placebo.
  - RESULTS:
    - – In those who received 1 mCi/kg, 72% had pain relief at 4 weeks ($p < 0.034$).
    - – 66% of responders at 4 weeks remained responsive at 16 weeks.
    - – Analgesic use ↓ in both the 0.5 and 1 mCi/kg groups, but statistical significance was only reached with 1 mCi/kg in comparison to placebo ($p > 0.093$).
    - – There was mild dose-related myelosuppression, with complete recovery by 8 weeks.
  - CONCLUSION:
    - – Single-dose 1 mCi/kg samarium-153 is effective in palliation of painful bone metastases.

Bisphosphonates

[Body JJ, *J Clin Oncol* **16**: 3890–3899, 1998]
[Saad F, *Eur Urol* **46**: 731–740, 2004]
[Eaton CL, *Cancer Treat Rev* **29**: 189–198, 2003]
[Garnero P, *Br J Cancer* **82**: 858–864, 2000]

- Have been primarily evaluated in patients with osteolytic bone metastases, such as multiple myeloma and breast cancer, but also have been shown to ↓ bone resorption in patients with osetoblastic metastases from prostate cancer.

- Limited effect on bone pain from prostate cancer.

- Clodronate.
  [Ernst DS, *J Clin Oncol* **21**: 3335–3342, 2003]
  - 209 patients with high-risk prostate cancer, bone metastases, and pain were randomized in a double-blind fashion to two groups.
    - – Group 1: mitoxantrone 12 mg/m^2, prednisone 5 mg b.i.d. and clodronate 1500 mg i.v. q 3 weeks × 10 cycles.
    - – Group 2: mitoxantrone/prednisone and placebo × 10 cycles.
  - RESULTS:
    - – 160 (77%) had mild pain and 24% had moderate pain upon study entry.

- Overall, there was no difference in palliative (pain + analgesic scores) response between groups (46% vs 39%; $p = 0.54$).
- On subgroup analysis, patients with baseline moderate pain had an improved palliative response (58% vs 26%; $p = 0.04$).
- There were no differences in overall quality-of-life scores, but there was significant improvement in the pain domain alone.
- No difference in survival (mean overall survival: 11 months).
  - CONCLUSIONS:
    - Clodronate does not improve palliative response, but may be beneficial in patients with moderate pain.

- [Dearnaley D, *J Natl Cancer Inst* **95**: 1300–1311, 2003]
  - 311 ♂ with hormone sensitive, metastatic bone disease were randomized in a double-blind fashion to two groups.
    - Group 1: clodronate 2080 mg/day for a maximum of 3 years.
    - Group 2: placebo for a maximum of 3 years.
  - RESULTS:
    - Non-significant but improved bone progression-free survival in the clodronate group (hazard ratio (HR) 0.79; $p = 0.08$).
    - Median time to progression: 23.6 vs 19.3 months.
    - No significant difference in overall survival (HR 0.80; $p = 0.082$).
    - Median overall survival: 37.1 vs 28.4 months.
    - Significant improvement in time to progression in a subgroup of patients who started clodronate within 6 weeks of starting hormone therapy (HR 0.48; 95% confidence interval 0.26 to 0.91).
  - CONCLUSIONS:
    - Adjuvant clodronate has a weak effect on altering the natural history of bone metastases.
    - The effect appears to be greatest when clodronate is started in close conjunction with the antiandrogen therapy.

- A placebo-controlled, multicenter trial evaluated pamidronate 90 mg i.v. q 3 weeks in symptomatic patients.
  [Small E, *J Clin Oncol* **21**: 4277–4284, 2003]
  - Slight ↓ in bone pain, but no effect on bone complications.

- More potent bisphosphonates have subsequently become available.

- Zoledronic acid.
  [Saad F, *J Natl Cancer Inst* **96**: 879–882, 2004]
  - 422 patients with high-risk prostate cancer and bone metastases were randomized to two groups.
    - Group 1: zoledronic acid 4 mg i.v. q 3 weeks × 15 months.
    - Group 2: placebo.

- Primary endpoint: skeletal-related events (SREs) defined as pathological fracture, spinal cord compression, radiation or surgery to bone, or any change in chemotherapy to treat bone pain.
- RESULTS:
  - Significant $\downarrow$ in the proportion of patients with SREs (38% vs 49% in placebo, $p = 0.029$), and an extended median time to first SRE (488 vs 321 days; $p = 0.009$).
  - On multiple-event analysis, zoledronic acid $\downarrow$ risk of developing SREs by 36% (HR 0.64; $p = 0.002$).
  - Zoledronic acid $\downarrow$ the mean annual incidence of SREs by 48% (0.77 vs 1.47; $p = 0.005$).
  - Bone pain was $\downarrow$ compared to placebo at 3, 9, 21, and 24 months.
- CONCLUSION:
  - Zoledronic acid 4 mg can $\downarrow$ the number of SREs and is not associated with undue toxicity or morbidity.

Side-effects of bisphosphonates

[Saunders Y, *Palliative Med* **18**: 418–431, 2004]

- Generally well-tolerated agents.

- Fever.
  - Especially with aminobisphosphonates, such as pamidronate and zoledronic acid.
  - Occurs in ~ 40% of patients.
  - May $\downarrow$ with prophylactic acetaminophen.

- Bone pain flare/arthalgias/myalgias.
  - < 10%, usually during the first 24 hours of parenteral administration.

- Hypocalcemia.
  - Generally mild, self-limited.
  - More common in the elderly.

- Nausea, dyspepsia.
  - Common with oral bisphosphonates, such as clodronate and alendronate.
  - Dose related.

- Renal insufficiency.
  [Markowitz GS, *Kidney Intl* **64**: 281–289, 2003]
  - Unknown mechanism; likely tubular injury.
  - Seen with all bisphosphonates.
  - $\downarrow$ risk with adequate hydration and prolonged infusion time.

- Ocular effects.
  [Fraunfelder FW, *N Engl J Med* **348**: 1187–1188, 2003]
  - Inflammatory reactions: uveitis, scleritis, conjunctivitis, and optic neuritis.
  - Occasionally vision threatening.
  - If the patient complains of ocular pain or visual disturbance, discontinue the bisphosphonate and consult an ophthalmologist.

- Jaw osteonecrosis.

Spinal cord compression

[Loblaw A, *J Clin Oncol* **23**: 2028–2037, 2005]
[Prasad D, *Lancet Oncol* **6**: 15–24, 2005]

- A common complication in patients with prostate cancer.
  - 90% of patients who die from prostate cancer have vertebral metastases.
  - Occurs in ~ 10–18% of cases.

- Pain and neurological deficits are key findings.
  - Back pain 83–95%.
    - Frequently precedes neurological deficits (by a mean of 8 weeks, but may be much longer).
    - May be sore on lying down if involving the epidural space.
    - Pain may evolve to be more radicular in distribution.
  - Motor deficits.
    - 60–85% of patients have weakness at the time of diagnosis.
    - Most apparent manifestation.
    - Up to 50% of patients are non-ambulatory when diagnosed.
  - Sensory deficits.
    - Often less pronounced than with motor dysfunction, but detectable in 40–90% of patients.
    - The sensory level is often several segments below the actual level of cord compression.
  - Bowel and bladder dysfunction.
    - Tend to occur late.
    - Urinary retention is the most common problem.
    - 50% of patients are catheter dependent at diagnosis.

- Need to maintain a high level of suspicion, with frequent neurological evaluations.

- Predictive factors of subclinical spinal cord compression in prostate cancer.
  [Bayley A, *Cancer* **92**: 303–310, 2001]
  - Extent of bone disease.
  - Duration of hormone therapy.
  - Back pain or analgesic use was <u>NOT</u> predictive.

Imaging

- MRI is the diagnostic test of choice to rule out significant cord or root compression.
  - It can be used to image the entire spine.
  - It has high soft tissue resolution and can reconstruct an image in several planes.
  - The entire spine must be imaged, not just the location to which neurological findings localize.

Management

1. Corticosteroids.
   - Have remained the mainstay of initial management.
   - There is no difference in outcome between high dose (dexamethasone 100 mg i.v. bolus) and moderate dose (dexamethasone 10 mg).
     [Vecht C, *Neurology* **39**: 1255–1257, 1989]
   - Maintenance corticosteroids are given after the initial bolus and maintained throughout the duration of radiation therapy; tapering of the dose begins following the completion of radiation therapy.

2. Neurosurgical assessment.
   [Sundaresan N, *J Clin Oncol* **13**: 2330–2335, 1995]
   [Loblaw AD, *J Clin Oncol* **16**: 1613–1624, 1998]
   - Relative indications:
     1. Spinal instability or boney compression.
     2. Neurological progression with radiation therapy.
     3. A site which has been irradiated previously.
   - The specific surgical procedure must be individualized according to the site and extent of disease. The approach and need for spinal stability will be case dependent.
   - The decision for surgery must also consider the acuity of spinal cord compression, neurological deficit, and patient comorbidity.
   - Patients may benefit from radiation therapy to site following surgery.

3. Radiotherapy.
   – Relative indications:
     1. No indications for surgery.
     2. Life expectancy < 3 months.
     3. > one level of simultaneous spinal cord compression.
     4. Patients with paraplegia of > 24 hours duration.
     5. Subclinical cord compression.
        [Bayley A, *Cancer* **92**: 303–310, 2001]

- Outcome is influenced by the presence of boney compression and ambulatory status prior to radiation therapy.

Soft tissue metastases

- Bone metastases are commonly seen in metastatic prostate cancer.

- Soft tissue metastases are rare in prostate cancer.

- Common sites of soft tissue metastases are lymph nodes (retroperitoneal, pelvic), liver, and lung.

- Soft tissue metastases are usually asymptomatic.

- Management is based on underlying disease characteristics.
  – See androgen deprivation treatment for hormone-sensitive disease (Chapter 21) and chemotherapy for hormone-refractory disease (Chapter 22).

- Response to chemotherapy (partial or complete remission) is infrequent in hormone-refractory metastatic disease.

- [Figg WD, *Cancer Invest* **14**: 513–517, 1996]
  - 177 consecutive ♂ following initial diagnosis of hormone-refractory prostate cancer underwent abdominal/pelvic computerized tomography (CT) scan, bone scan, and prostate-specific antigen (PSA) testing.
  - RESULTS:
    – 34 ♂ (19.2%) had measurable lesions (≥ 2 cm) on CT scan compatible with metastatic disease.
    – Of the ♂ with measurable lesions, 29/34 (85.3%) had retroperitoneal and/or pelvic adenopathy; 5 ♂ (14.7%) had measurable lesions in the liver.
    – Other sites of metastatic disease were detected in < 1% of the ♂ receiving scans.

- All ♂ had bone-scan abnormalities compatible with metastatic disease.
- The mean PSA concentration was <u>not</u> different in those patients with soft tissue disease as compared with those without soft tissue involvement.
- There was no correlation between PSA concentration and the presence or absence of measurable soft tissue disease.

- [Petrylak D, *N Engl J Med* **351**: 1513–1520, 2004]
  - 770 ♂ with high-risk prostate cancer were randomized.
    - Group I (DE): docetaxel and estramustine.
    - Group II (MP): mitoxantrone and prednisone.
  - PATIENT CHARACTERISTICS:
    - Bone metastasis.
      - Group I (DE): 84%.
      - Group II (MP): 88%.
    - Soft tissue metastases (visceral disease).
      - Lymph node: 24% → DE, 26% → MP.
      - Liver: 8% → DE, 9% → MP.
      - Lung: 10% in both DE and MP.
  - RESULTS:
    - Partial response in measurable disease.
      - Group I (DE): 17%.
      - Group II (MP): 10%.

- [Tannock I, *N Engl J Med* **351**: 1502–1512, 2004]
  - 1006 ♂ with high-risk prostate cancer were randomized.
    - Group I (D3W): docetaxel q 3 weeks.
    - Group II (DW): docetaxel q week.
    - Group III (M): mitoxantrone q 3 weeks.
  - PATIENT CHARACTERISTICS:
    - All patients received prednisone.
    - Bone metastasis: 90%, D3W; 91%, DW; 92%, M.
    - Soft tissue metastases (visceral disease): 22%, D3W; 24%, DW; 22% M.
  - RESULTS:
    - Partial response in measurable disease.
      - Group I (D3W): 12%.
      - Group II (DW): 8%.
      - Group III (M): 7%.

21

Endocrine therapy for metastatic prostate cancer

- Androgenic stimuli are needed for both malignant transformation and growth of prostate tissue.
- The testes produce ~ 90% of total circulating testosterone.
- The adrenal glands produce ~ 10% of the remaining testosterone.
- 24–30 months is the median survival time, depending on the extent of disease at presentation.
- Testosterone < 10 ng/ml is castrate level.
- ~ 80% respond to initial hormone therapy, and all patients later progress to androgen independence.
  [Grayhack JT, *Cancer* **60**: 589–601, 1987]

Androgen-deprivation therapy

- The primary therapeutic approach for metastatic prostate cancer.
- Alleviates bone pain in ~ 80–90% of ♂.
- ↓ prostate-specific antigen (PSA) levels, soft tissue, and bone disease.
- Most ♂ develop hormone-refractory disease within 18–24 months.
  - Hormone-refractory disease refers to disease progression with castrate levels of testosterone.
- Available methods of androgen-deprivation therapy (ADT).
  - Surgical.
    - Bilateral orchiectomy.

- Medical.
  - Leuteinizing hormone releasing hormone (LHRH) agonists (leuprolide, goserelin, buserelin).
  - LHRH antagonists (abarelix).
  - Androgen antagonists.
    - Non-steroidal (flutamide, bicalutamide, nilutamide).
    - Steroidal (cyproterone acetate).
  - Complete androgen blockade (CAB) → LHRH agonists with an androgen antagonist.
  - Progesterone agents (megestrol acetate).

Orchiectomy

- Relatively simple procedure with minor surgical risks.
- ↓ utilization given its psychological impact, other viable medical alternatives, and irreversibility.
- ↓ total testosterone ~ 90%.
- Compliance is not an issue.
- SIDE-EFFECTS:
  - Hot flashes (50%), psychologic effects, gynecomastia.
- No flare response.
- Least costly in long run.

Leuteinizing hormone releasing hormone agonists

- Goserelin (Zoladex) 10.8 mg s.c. q 12 weeks.
- Leuprolide (Lupron) 7.5 mg s.c. q 28 days or 22.5 mg s.c. q 12 weeks or 30 mg s.c. q 16 weeks.
- Buserelin (Suprefact) 6.6 mg s.c. q 60 days or 9.9 mg s.c. q 90 days.
- Leads to castration levels within 3 weeks.
- SIDE-EFFECTS:
  - Hot flashes (60%), sexual dysfunction (100%), ↓ erections (100%), gynecomastia, osteopenia, muscle loss, weight gain, and depression.
- Flare response can occur due to a testosterone surge in the first 4 weeks of LHRH agonists.

- Block with androgen antagonist prior to or when starting therapy and up to 4 weeks.

- Expensive.

Leuteinizing hormone releasing hormone antagonists

- Abarelix (Plenaxis) 100 mg i.m. in buttock on days 1, 15, and 29, and then q 4 weeks.

- No initial flare.

- Indicated for impending cord compression or other uncommon clinical scenarios where LHRH agonists are contraindicated. Theoretical advantage only.

- SIDE-EFFECTS:
  - Back pain, bladder pain, breast enlargement, osteopenia.

- ~ 4% risk of anaphylaxis.

- Expensive.

Androgen antagonists (anti-androgens)

- Non-steroidal.
  - Bicalutamide (Casodex) 50 mg p.o. q day.
  - Flutamide (Eulexin) 250 mg p.o. t.i.d.
  - Nilutamide (Nilandron) 300 mg p.o. q day × 30 days, then 150 mg p.o. q day.
  - SIDE-EFFECTS:
    - ↑ Liver function tests (LFTs), mild nausea, mild skin rash, impotence, gynecomastia, hot flashes, vertigo, night blindness (nilutamide), interstitial pneumonitis (nilutamide, black box warning), diarrhea (flutamide).

- Steroidal.
  - Cyproterone acetate (Cyprostat) 100–200 mg 2–4 tablets p.o. q day divided into 2–3 doses, or 300 mg (3 ml) i.m. q week. Not used in the USA.
  - SIDE-EFFECTS:
    - ↑ LFTs, thrombosis, gynecomastia, hot flashes, nausea, impotence, vertigo, weight gain.

- **American Society of Clinical Oncology (ASCO) recommendations for the initial hormonal management of androgen-sensitive meta-**

static, recurrent, or progressive prostate cancer.
[Andrew J, *Clin Oncol* **22**(14): 2927–2941, 2004]
- 10 randomized, controlled trials, 6 systematic reviews, and 1 Markov model were available to inform the guidelines.
- Bilateral orchiectomy or LHRH agonists are the recommended initial treatments.
- Non-steroidal anti-androgen therapy may be discussed as an alternative, but steroidal anti-androgens should not be offered as monotherapy.
- ♂ willing to accept the ↑ toxicity of CAB for a small benefit in survival should be offered non-steroidal anti-androgen therapy in addition to castrate therapy.
- Shared decision-making between ♂ and physicians is necessary for optimum use of ADT.

- **Comparing LHRH agonists with orchiectomy or diethylstilbestrol, and to compare anti-androgens with any of these three alternatives.**
[Seidenfeld J, *Ann Intern Med* **132**: 566–577, 2000]
  - Meta-analysis of 24 trials involving more than 6,600 ♂.
    - 10 trials of LHRH agonists involving 1,908 ♂ reported no significant difference in overall survival (OS).
    - The hazard ratio (HR) showed LHRH agonists to be essentially equivalent to orchiectomy (HR 1.262; 95% confidence interval (CI) 0.915 to 1.386).
  - 8 trials involving 2,717 ♂ suggest that non-steroidal anti-androgens as monotherapy are associated with ↓ OS.
  - CONCLUSION:
    - All provide similar efficacy as monotherapy, except anti-androgens which may be slightly inferior.

Complete androgen blockade

- LHRH agonists block testicular androgens.

- Anti-androgens block adrenal androgens.

- Although commonly used, the benefit of CAB over monotherapy remains uncertain despite several trials.

Complete androgen blockade versus monotherapy

- 3 randomized trials suggest survival benefit for CAB.

- Several meta-analyses suggest a small survival benefit for CAB over monotherapy.

- The largest US intergroup trial did not find any benefit of CAB.

- **Bilateral orchiectomy with or without flutamide for metastatic prostate cancer.**
  [Eisenberger MA, *N Engl J Med* **339**(15):1036–1042, 1998]
  - 1,387 ♂ were enrolled in the trial.
    - Group I: 700 ♂ randomly assigned to the flutamide group.
    - Group II: 687 ♂ randomly assigned to the placebo group.
  - RESULTS:
    - No significant difference in OS ($p = 0.14$).
  - SIDE-EFFECTS:
    - Minimal; the only notable differences between the groups were the greater rates of diarrhea and anemia with flutamide.
  - CONCLUSION:
    - The addition of flutamide to bilateral orchiectomy did not result in a clinically meaningful improvement in survival.

- **Meta-analysis of monotherapy compared with CAB for patients with advanced prostate carcinoma.**
  [Samson DJ, *Cancer* **95**(2): 361–376, 2002]
  - 21 trials compared survival after monotherapy vs CAB ($n = 6,871$ ♂).
  - RESULTS:
    - No statistically significant difference in survival at 2 years. (20 trials; HR 0.970; 95% CI 0.866 to 1.087).
    - Statistically significant difference in survival at 5 years that favored CAB (10 trials; HR 0.871; 95% CI 0.805 to 0.942).
  - SIDE-EFFECT:
    - Withdrawal from therapy occurred more often with CAB.

- **Maximum androgen blockade in advanced prostate cancer: an overview of randomized trials.**
  [Prostate Cancer Trialists' Collaborative Group, *Lancet* **355**(9214): 1491–1498, 2000]
  - Androgen suppression by surgery or drugs vs CAB.
  - Meta-analysis of 27 randomized trials of 8,275 ♂.
  - Follow-up ~ 5 years.
  - RESULTS:
    - 5-year survival → 25.4% vs 23.6% for CAB and androgen suppression, respectively.
  - CONCLUSION:
    - In advanced prostate cancer, addition of an anti-androgen to

androgen suppression improved the 5-year survival by about 2–3%.

Early versus deferred androgen-deprivation therapy

- **ASCO recommendations for the initial hormone management of androgen-sensitive metastatic, recurrent, or progressive prostate cancer.**
  [Loblaw AD, *J Clin Oncol* **22**(14): 2927–2941, 2004]
  - No specific recommendations can be issued.
  - A discussion about the pros and cons of early vs deferred therapy should occur between ♂ and practitioner.
  - Anti-androgen monotherapy is not recommended.
  - ♂ may be followed clinically and started on ADT once symptoms of locally progressive or metastatic disease present.
  - Early treatment with LHRH agonists confers a small but statistically significant survival advantage, and significant improvements in progression-free survival that are durable up to 10 years of follow-up.
  - These results are based on a systematic review of trials that did not select a cohort of ♂ who progressed post-treatment, on surveillance, or who had metastatic disease on presentation.
  - Treatment was most cost-effective when started after the onset of symptoms.

Intermittent androgen suppression

- **Limited phase II data.**
- **3 current phase III trials evaluating intermittent androgen suppression (IAS).**
  - European EC507 comparing IAS with CAB.
  - Southwest Oncology Group (SWOG) S9346 (INT-0162) evaluating the equivalence of IAS and CAB.
  - National Cancer Institute of Canada (NCIC) PR.7 (JPR7) comparing the OS with IAS to the OS with continuous suppression.
- **Should still be considered experimental.**
- **Selected phase II data.**
  [Goldenberg SL, *Mol Urol* **3**: 287–292, 1999]
  - 87 ♂ treated with IAS.

- CAB was initiated and held once the PSA nadir occurred.
- CAB restarted when PSA ↑ to 10–20 ng/ml.
- RESULTS:
  - Average time off therapy per cycle:
    - 1–15 months: 54%.
    - 2–10 months: 48%.
    - 3–8 months: 45%.
    - 4–7 months: 40%.
- CONCLUSION:
  - IAS provides improved quality of life, with a lower cost and without a negative impact on outcome.

- A similar trial demonstrated a median OS of 166 weeks. [Goldenberg SL, *Urology* **45**: 839–844, 1995]

- Several other trials have demonstrated similar findings.

- Quality of life trial for IAS. [Grossfeld GD, *Urology* **58**: 240–245, 2001]
  - 10 ♂ evaluated.
  - RESULTS:
    - All ♂ experienced significant improvements in fatigue, vitality, and sexual function.

Androgen antagonist addition

- There is an ~ 10% ↑ response rate by adding an androgen antagonist once disease has progressed on castrate therapy.

Androgen antagonist subtraction (androgen withdrawal)

- Removal of an androgen antagonist once disease progresses on CAB may cause a paradoxical shrinkage of disease, PSA, and symptoms in ~ 25% of ♂.

- The initial step once failing on CAB.

Other endocrine therapy used in prostate cancer

- **Megestrol acetate (Megace).**
  - 160 mg p.o. q day.

- SIDE-EFFECTS:
  - Mild alopecia, ↑ LFTs, fluid retention, intrahepatic cholestasis, thromboembolism.

- **Phase III trial comparing orchiectomy + cyproterone acetate and low-dose diethylstilbestrol in the management of metastatic prostate cancer.**
  [Robinson MR, *Eur Urol* **28**(4): 273–283, 1995]
  - 328 eligible ♂ followed up for a median of 4 years.
  - RESULTS:
    - No difference in time to metastatic progression or OS between the treatment groups.
  - SIDE-EFFECT:
    - The cardiovascular toxicity of diethylstilbestrol resulted in more deaths than did orchiectomy alone.

- **Ketoconazole (Nizoral).**
  - Used for adrenal androgen suppression.
  - Start at 200 mg p.o. t.i.d. and ↑ to 400 mg p.o. t.i.d.
  - SIDE-EFFECT:
    - Liver toxicity.
  - Monitor LFTs.

- **Aminoglutethimide (Cytadren).**
  - Used for adrenal androgen suppression.
  - 125–250 mg p.o. q.i.d.
  - Caution with adrenal insufficiency.
  - Should be given with hydrocortisone 100 mg/day in divided doses × 2 weeks, then 40 mg in divided doses.
  - SIDE-EFFECTS:
    - Weakness, fever, rash.

- **Hydrocortisone.**
  - 20 mg p.o. b.i.d.
  - Significant pain relief.
  - Minor objective tumor response.
  - SIDE-EFFECTS:
    - Edema, hyperglycemia, proximal muscle weakness, skin changes, depression, gastrointestinal disturbances.

Bone mineralization management

- **Prevention of osteoporosis in ♂ undergoing treatment with an LHRH agonist.**

[Smith MR, *N Engl J Med* **345**(13): 948–955, 2001]

- Open-label study, with 47 randomly assigned ♂ with advanced or recurrent prostate cancer.
- No bone metastases.
  - Group I: leuprolide alone.
  - Group II: leuprolide + pamidronate 60 mg i.v. q 12 weeks.
- RESULTS:
  - The mean bone mineral density did not change significantly at any skeletal site in ♂ treated with both leuprolide + pamidronate.
- CONCLUSION:
  - Pamidronate prevents bone loss in the hip and lumbar spine in ♂ receiving treatment for prostate cancer with LHRH agonists.

- **Effect of zoledronic acid on bone mineral density during ADT for non-metastatic prostate cancer.**
  [Smith MR, *J Urol* **169**(6): 2008–2012, 2003]
  - Multicenter, double-blind, randomized, placebo-controlled clinical trial.
  - 106 ♂ enrolled to one of two groups.
    - Group I: zoledronic acid 4 mg i.v. q 3 months for 1 year.
    - Group II: placebo.
  - The primary efficacy variable was the percentage change from baseline to 1 year in bone mineral density of the lumbar spine as measured by dual-energy x-ray absorptiometry.
  - RESULTS:
    - Mean bone mineral density in the lumbar spine ↑ by 5.6% in group I vs a ↓ of 2.2% for group II ($p < 0.001$).
  - CONCLUSION:
    - Zoledronic acid ↑ bone mineral density in the hip and spine during ADT for non-metastatic prostate cancer.

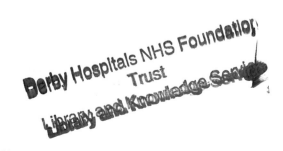

22

Chemotherapy in hormone-refractory prostate cancer

[Kent EC, *Urology* **62** (Suppl 6B): 134–140, 2003]
[Bhandari MS, *Eur J Cancer* **41**: 941–953, 2005]
[Petryluk D, *Urology* **65** (Suppl5A): 3–8, 2005]

- Historically ♂ were designated 'hormone-refractory' if they simply progressed while on primary hormone therapy.

- It became evident that some of these 'hormone-refractory' ♂ may still respond to secondary hormonal maneuvers, such as corticosteriods, ketoconazole, or antiandrogen withdrawal.

- In 1999, the PSA Working Group published three requirements to establish hormone-refractory prostate cancer (HRPC).
  [Bubley GJ, *J Clin Oncol* **17**: 3461–3467, 1999]
  1. Documented progressive disease.
  2. Serum testosterone within the castrate range.
  3. Adequate trial of antiandrogen withdrawal.

- In spite of disease progression, <u>castration should be maintained</u> to optimize outcome.

- Measurable disease is only present in 20–30% of cases, and therefore response evaluation usually involves prostate-specific antigen (PSA) (biochemical) response, and clinical response, including quality of life, time to progression, and overall survival.

- Once hormone-refractory status is established:
  - Time to progression → ~ 10–16 months.
  - Overall survival → ~ 16–24 months.

- Until recently, the goal of chemotherapy was improved palliation of symptoms and improved quality of life.
  - No previous therapy had been shown to favorably impact on survival.

Prognostic factors in hormone-refractory prostate cancer

[Halabi S, *J Clin Oncol* **21**: 1232–1237, 2003]
[Smaletz O, *J Clin Oncol* **20**: 3972–3982, 2002]

- A wide range in outcome in ♂ with HRPC has been reported.

- With the use of PSA as a widely accepted endpoint, there is a need to stratify HRPC patients into at least three subcategories:
  1. PSA-only disease.
  2. Increasing PSA with stable metastatic disease.
  3. Increasing PSA with objective progression.

- The presence or absence of symptoms is also a useful determinant for the institution of therapy.

- A variety of independent prognostic factors has been described.
  - Age.
  - Performance status.
  - Initial Gleason score.
  - Initial PSA.
  - Prior response to hormone therapy.
  - Weight loss.
  - Extent of bone disease.
  - Presence or absence of soft tissue disease.
  - Hemoglobin.
  - Lactate dehydrogenase.
  - Alkaline phosphatase.
  - PSA velocity.
  - PSA response to therapy.

Historical overview of chemotherapy in hormone-refractory prostate cancer

- In the pre-taxane era, no single agent had tumor activity beyond 15%.

- Prior to the 1990s, ♂ with symptomatic HRPC were treated with low-dose corticosteroids, resulting in a 10–15% improvement in pain and other quality-of-life measures.

- 161 ♂ with symptomatic HRPC were randomized in a clinical trial.
  [Tannock I, *J Clin Oncol* **114**: 1756–1764, 1996]
  - Group I: prednisone 5 mg p.o. b.i.d. alone.
  - Group II: mitoxantrone 12 mg/m² + prednisone 5 mg p.o. b.i.d.
  - Primary response defined → 2 point ↓ in pain-intensity scale with no ↑ in analgesics.
  - RESULTS:
    - Group II had 29% with a primary palliative response compared with 12% in the prednisone alone group ($p = 0.01$).
    - Response duration was longer in group II (43 vs 18 weeks, $p < 0.0001$).
    - No difference in survival.

- Cancer and Leukemia Group B (CALGB) 9182.
  [Kantoff PW, *J Clin Oncol* **17**: 2506–2513, 1999]
  - Similar design to the Tannock study.
  - 242 ♂ randomized.
    - Group I: hydrocortisone 40 mg/day.
    - Group II: mitoxantrone 14 mg/m² + hydrocortisone 40 mg/day.
  - RESULTS:
    - No difference in survival, but some improvement in time to disease progression (3.7 vs 2.3 months, $p = 0.025$).

Consequently:
Mitoxantrone in combination with low-dose prednisone became the standard of care for symptomatic HRPC.

Single-agent docetaxel

[Crown J, *Anticancer Drug* **10**(Suppl 1): S19–S24, 1999]
[Engels F, *Eur J Cancer* **41**: 1117–1126, 2005]

- Antimicrotubule agent.

- Initially extracted from the bark of the Pacific yew (*Taxus brevifolia*) and from the European yew (*Taxus baccata*).

- Phase II studies in the 1990s showed activity as a single agent in weekly and q 3 weeks schedules.
  [Piscus J, *Semin Oncol* **26**(5 Suppl 14): 14–18, 1999]
  [Gravis G, *Cancer* **98**(8): 1627–1634, 2003]
  [Ferrero J, *Oncology* **66**(4): 281–287, 2004]
  - > 50% PSA response rates and tumor response rates of 40% were observed.

- Median survival range → 9–27 months.
- < hematological toxicity was observed with the weekly schedules.

Randomized trials of docetaxel

- TAX 327.
  [Tannock I, *N Engl J Med* **351**: 1502–1512, 2004]
  - 1006 ♂ with progressive HRPC, no prior chemotherapy.
  - Stable level of pain for 7 days prior to randomization.
    - Group I: docetaxel 75 mg/m^2 q 3 weeks + prednisone 5 mg b.i.d.
    - Group II: docetaxel 30 mg/m^2 for 5 of 6 weeks + prednisone 5 mg b.i.d.
    - Group III: mitoxantrone 12 mg/m^2 q 3 weeks + prednisone 5 mg b.i.d.
  - Median age: 68 years.
  - Characteristics.
    - 90% bone disease.
    - 24% visceral disease.
    - Most were eligible because of progression on bone scan or PSA.
    - 45% pain at baseline.
  - RESULTS:

Endpoint	Group I	Group II	Group III
Evaluable (n)	141	134	137
Response rate (%)	12	8	7
p	0.1	0.5	
Overall survival (months)	18.9	17.3	16.4
Hazard ratio	0.76	0.91	
p	0.0009	0.3	
PSA response	45	48	32
p	0.0005	< 0.00001	
Pain response rate:			
Evaluable (n)	153	154	157
Response rate (%)	35	31	22
p	0.01	0.07	

  - ~ 25% of ♂ receiving docetaxel had a significant improvement in quality of life compared to those receiving mitoxantrone.
  - Treatment in all groups was well tolerated.

- Febrile neutropenia and infections were uncommon.
- Southwest Oncology Group (SWOG) 9916.
  [Petrylak D, *N Engl J Med* **351:** 1513–1520, 2004]
  - 770 ♂ with progressive, metastatic HRPC (similar to the TAX 327 study).
  - Randomized to two groups of treatment given in 21-day cycles:
  - Group I: estramustine 280 mg p.o. t.i.d. on days 1–5 +:
    - docetaxel 60 mg/m^2 i.v. on day 2
    - prednisone 5 mg p.o. b.i.d. continuously.
    - (Note: all patients received warfarin 2 mg q day + aspirin 325 mg q day in estramustine group.)
  - Group II: mitoxantrone 12 mg/m^2 i.v. q 21 days.
    - Prednisone 5 mg p.o. b.i.d. continuously.
- RESULTS:

Endpoint	Group I	Group II
Tumor response rate (%)	17	11
Evaluable (*n*)	103	93
p	0.15	
Overall survival (months)	18	16
Hazard ratio	0.80	
p	0.01	
Progression-free survival (months)	6	3
Hazard ratio	0.73	
p	< 0.0001	
PSA response rate (%)	50	27
p	< 0.0001	

- SIDE-EFFECTS:
  - Higher rates of toxicity were seen with docetaxel/estramustine, yet there was no difference in toxic death rates or the rate of study discontinuation.

TAX 327 and SWOG 9916 taken together

- Docetaxel q 3 weeks with low-dose prednisone represents the new standard of care for HRPC.

- Docetaxel is superior to mitoxantrone in survival, PSA response, tumor response, pain control, and quality of life.

- Although no direct comparative studies of docetaxel with or without estramustine have been performed, there appeared to be no improvement in survival or response rates with estamustine in the SWOG 9916 compared to docetaxel alone in TAX 327.

- Both approved and investigational agents are currently being studied in combination with docetaxel.

Toxicity of docetaxel

[Engels F, *Eur J Cancer* **41**: 1117–1126, 2005]

- Docetaxel (Taxotere) given in q 3-week cycles at a dose of 60–75 mg/m^2.

- Neutropenia: dose limiting.
  - Nadir develops on day 4–7.

- Fatigue and asthenia most common (5–20% incidence).

- Edema.
  - Usually involves the periphery and the pleural space (not cardiac).
  - Common, especially (> 80%) if not premedicated with corticosteroids (e.g. dexamethasone 8 mg p.o. b.i.d. × 3 days beginning 24 hours prior to treatment).

- Hypersensitivity reactions common.
  - Recommend routine corticosteroid prophylaxis.

- Skin toxicity.
  - Nail changes common: onycholysis uncommon.
  - May be prevented by placing finger and toe nails in iced water during infusion.
  - Maculopapular eruption may occur, especially with first cycle.

- Neurotoxicity.
  - Numbness and weakness.
  - Dysaestheisa may occur.
  - Tends to be cumulative and slowly reversible.
  - Pyridoxine may be helpful.

- Alopecia.
  - Occurs in ~ 80%.

- Hyperlacrimation.
  - Usually mild, but can be bothersome.

- Results from canalicular/nasolacrimal duct stenosis.
- Associated with prolonged therapy (> 1000 mg cumulative dose).
- May require ophthalmologic evaluation if persistent or severe.

- Nausea and diarrhea.
  - Can occur in ~ 40%.
  - ↓ with corticosteroid prophylaxis and antiemetic agents.

- Mucositis.
  - Usually mild; parallels neutropenia.

Estramustine

- Estramustine (Emcyt): nor-nitrogen mustard carbamate derivative of estradiol-17β-phosphate,

- Interrupts microtubule assembly.

- Synergistic with other microtubule-targeting agents, such as taxanes and vinca alkaloids.

- Oral agent:
  - Dose: 10–14 mg/m^2 q day in 3 divided doses.
  - Should not be taken with milk or calcium-containing drugs, as calcium interferes with absorption.

- SIDE-EFFECTS:
  - Nausea.
    - Commonly seen soon after starting treatment; lessens with continued use.
  - ↑ in lactate dehydrogenase and aspartate transaminase is common.
  - Fluid retention common; avoid use in patients with congestive heart failure or pre-existing cardiac disease.
  - Gynecomastia and breast tenderness are common.
  - Thromboembolic disease: risk is ↑ when given with concurrent chemotherapy.
    - Anticoagulant prophylaxis with warfarin (Coumadin) and aspirin is recommended with continued use.

- Previously used as a single agent in symptomatic HRPC.

- Synergistic with docetaxel 70 mg/m^2 q 3 weeks in phase II testing.
  [Kreis W, *Ann Oncol* **10**: 33–38, 1999]
  [Petrylak DP, *Semin Oncol* **26**(Suppl 17): 28–33, 1999]
  [Savarese DM, *J Clin Oncol* **22**: 2532–2539, 2001]

- 50% PSA ↓: 45–74%.
- Response in measurable disease: 20–50%.
- Median survival: 13–20 months.
- HOWEVER in SWOG 9916, estramustine did not appear to add any beneficial effect on survival and response rates, as was seen in the docetaxel q 3 weeks group in TAX 327.

Docetaxel-refractory patients

- No chemotherapeutic agent has yet shown benefit in patients who progress following docetaxel.

- Ongoing studies.
  - AP23573 in patients with taxane-resistant, androgen-independent prostate cancer (ARAID Pharmaceuticals Inc.).
  - Study of Irofulven (hydroxymethylacylfulvene) in patients with HRPC (MGI Pharma).
  - Satraplatin in HRPC patients previously treated with one cytotoxic chemotherapy regimen (GPC-Biotech).

Ongoing clinical trials in hormone-refractory prostate cancer

[Bhandri MS, *Eur J Cancer* **41**: 941–953, 2005]
[Strother JM, *Eur J Cancer* **41**: 954–964, 2005]

- Epothilones.
  - Induce microtubule stabilization, leading to mitotic arrest at G2/M.
  - BMS-247550.
  - [Hussain M, *Proc Am Soc Clin Oncol* **23**: 383 (abstract 4510), 2004]
    - Phase II study in 41 ♂.
    - PSA response rate: 16/41 (41%).
    - Measurable response rate: 3/19 (16%).
    - Progression-free survival: 8 months.
  - [Kelly WK, *Proc Am Soc Clin Oncol* **23**: 383 (abstract 4509), 2004]
    - Randomized, phase II study of BMS-247550 with (BE) or without estramustine (B) in 92 chemotherapy-naive patients.
    - PSA response: BE 22/32 (69%); B 18/32 (56%).
    - Measurable response rate: BE 8/18 (44%); B 6/26 (23%).
  - Preclinical evidence for non-cross-resistance with docetaxel → possible second-line agent.

- On-going study.
  - Eastern Cooperative Oncology Group (ECOG) E3803.
  - Phase II study of ixabepilone q 3 or 4 weeks in patients with metastatic HRPC.

- Thalidomide.
  - Anti-angiogenic: exact mechanism is unclear → possible through vascular endothelial growth factor (VEGF) inhibition.
  - [Figg WD, *Clin Cancer Res* **7**: 1888–1893, 2001]
    - Randomized, phase II study of 63 patients to receive either low-dose thalidomide (200 mg/day) or high-dose thalidomide (dose escalation to the maximum tolerated dose or 1200 mg).
    - Only 13 patients were treated in the high-dose group – poorly tolerated.
    - In the low-dose group, PSA response: 9/50 (15%).
  - [Dahut WL, *J Clin Oncol* **22**: 2532–2539, 2004]
    - Randomized, phase II trial of docetaxel (D) with or without thalidomide (T) 200 mg/day in 53 chemotherapy-naive patients.
    - PSA response: DT 19/36 (53%); D 6/17 (35%).
    - Progression-free survival: DT, 5.9 months; D, 3.7 months.
    - Overall survival (at 18 months): DT, 68%; D, 43%.
  - Ongoing studies.
    - NCI-V01-1681: phase II study of docetaxel, estramustine, and thalidomide.
    - NCI-04-C-0132: phase II study of docetaxel, estramustine, and thalidomide.
    - Also, current studies with thalidomide analogues, such as lenalidomide (Revimid).

- Bevacizumab (Avastin).
  - Recombinant anti-VEGF monoclonal antibody.
  - Used in combination with docetaxel.
  - CALGB 90006.
    [Picus J, *Proc Am Soc Clin Oncol* **22**: 393 (abstract 1578), 2003]
    - Phase II study of bevacizumab with docetaxel and estramustine in 79 patients with chemotherapy-naive HRPC.
    - Preliminary results only.
      - PSA response rate: 13/20 (65%).
      - Measurable tumor response: 9/17 (53%).

- Atrasentan.
  - Selective endothelial receptor antagonist.
  - Well tolerated at 10 mg/day p.o.

- [Carducci MA, *J Clin Oncol* **21**: 679–689, 2003]
  Randomized, phase II, placebo-controlled trial in 288 patients
  with asymptomatic metastatic HRPC, comparing atrasentan (A)
  2.5 mg/day and 10 mg/day with placebo (P).
  - Mean time to PSA progression:
    - A 10 mg, 155 days; P, 71 days; $p = 0.002$.
  - Median time to progression (in evaluable patients):
    - A 10 mg, 196 days; P, 129 days; $p = 0.021$.
  - SIDE-EFFECTS:
    - Headache, peripheral edema, rhinitis.
- [Carducci MA, *Proc Am Soc Clin Oncol* **23**: 384 (abstract 4508), 2004]
  Phase III, placebo-controlled study of atrasentan 10 mg/day in 809
  patients with metastatic HRPC.
  - Preliminary results:
    - Time to clinical/radiologic progression: hazard ratio 1.14
      (95% CI 0.98 to 1.34; $p = 0.091$).
    - Time to PSA progression: hazard ratio 1.78 (95% CI 1.34 to
      2.37; $p < 0.001$).
    - No survival data as yet.
- Planned phase III study of docetaxel/prednisone with and without
  atrasentan (SWOG-S0421).

- Bcl-2 antisense.
  - Bcl-2 protein is overexpressed in HRPC cells and confers resist-
    ance to apoptosis.
  - G3139 (oblimersen): antisense oligonucleotide directed to first 6
    codons of human Bcl-2 mRNA.
  - [Chi KN, *Proc Am Soc Clin Oncol* **22**: 393 (abstract 1580), 2003]
    Phase II trial of G3139 7 mg/kg q day continuous i.v. infusion on
    days 1–8 in combination with docetaxel 75 mg/m² i.v. on day 6 in
    29 ♂ with metastatic HRPC.
    - RESULTS:
      - PSA response rate: 15/31 (48%).
      - Measurable response rate: 4/15 (27%).
  - Ongoing study:
    - EORTC 30021: docetaxel with or without oblimersen in HRPC.

- Calcitriol (DN101).
  - Active metabolite of vitamin D; inhibits growth associated with
    cell-cycle arrest, induces apoptosis, and possible synergy with
    cytotoxic agents.
  - [Beer TM, *J Clin Oncol* **21**: 123–128, 2003]
    Phase II study of DN101 0.5 μ/kg p.o. on day 1 and docetaxel

36 mg/m^2 on day 2, repeated weekly for 6 or 8 weeks in 37 patients with metastatic HRPC.
- PSA response: 30/37 (81%).
- Measurable tumor response: 8/15 (53%).
- Median time to progression: 11.4 months.
- Median survival: 19.5 months.

- ASCENT trial.
  [Beer TM, *Proc Am Soc Clin Oncol* **24**: 382 (abstract 4516), 2005]
  - Phase III, placebo-controlled trial of DN101 and docetaxel 36 mg/m^2 for 3 or 4 weeks in 809 ♂ with metastatic HRPC.
  - Interim analysis at median follow-up of 8 months.
  - RESULTS:
    - 250 chemotherapy-naive patients randomized to docetaxel + oral DN101 (DN) or placebo (P).
    - PSA response (primary endpoint): DN, 58%; P, 49%; not significant.
    - Measurable response rate: DN, 13/46 (28%); P, 11/56 (20%); not significant.
    - Median survival (secondary endpoint): DN, 23.5 months; P, 16.4 months (HR 0.70, $p = 0.07$).

- Other multicenter clinical trials in HRPC.
  - GVAX vaccine for prostate cancer vs docetaxel and prednisone in patients with metastatic HRPC (Cell Genesys Inc.).
  - APC8015 (Provenge) in treating patients with asymptomatic metastatic androgen-independent prostate cancer (Denreon Corp./NCI).
  - Docetaxel with or without imatinib mesylate in treating patients with androgen-independent prostate cancer and bone metastases (NCI_Pharma. PI: Drs Paul Matthew, Chris Logothetis).
  - Docetaxel with or without dimethylxanthenone acetic acid (AS1404) in treating patients with metastatic prostate cancer that did not respond to previous hormone therapy (Antisoma Research Ltd. PI: Dr Miroslav Ravic).
  - Sorafenib in treating patients with metastatic or recurrent prostate cancer (NCIC IND 167. PI: K. Chi).

23

Investigational agents

New cytotoxic agents

Epothilone (EPO906) and epothilone analogue ixabepilone (BMS-247550)

[Hussain A, *Proc Am Soc Clin Oncol* **23**: 396 (abstract 4565), 2004]
[Kelly WK, *Proc Am Soc Clin Oncol* **23**: 383 (abstract 4510), 2004]

- Third-generation anti-microtubule agents.

- Mechanism of action is microtubular stabilization, resulting in mitotic arrest in the G2/M phase.

- Phase II trials for EPO906 showed 22% prostate-specific antigen (PSA) response in 37 patients with previously treated hormone-refractory prostate cancer (HRPC).

- Ixabepilone (BMS-247550) is active in chemotherapy-naive patients with metastatic HRPC.

- Southwest Oncology Group (SWOG) 0111.
  [Hussain A, *J Clin Oncol* **34**: 8724–8729, 2005]
  - Randomized, phase II study in 92 chemotherapy-naive patients: 56% PSA and 23% measurable disease response for BMS-247550 alone, and 69% PSA and 44% measurable disease response rates in combination with estramustine.
  - RESULTS:
    - 48 patients: 33% confirmed PSA responses.
    - 72% of responders had declines > 80%.

- Median progression-free survival → 6 months.
- Median survival → 18 months.
- SIDE-EFFECTS:
  - Gastrointestinal (EPO906).
  - Leukopenia/neutropenia (grade 4).
  - Sensory neuropathy (grade 3).
  - Fatigue.
  - Flu-like symptoms.

Irofulven

[Senzer N, *Am J Clin Oncol* **28**(1): 36–42, 2005]

- Irofulven (hydroxymethylacylfulvene) is a novel DNA-binding agent that induces apoptosis independent of *p53* or *p21* status with cytotoxicity in drug-resistant cell lines.

- Phase II trial of 42 patients with chemotherapy-naive HRPC demonstrated PSA stability in 64% and PSA response in 13%.
  - SIDE-EFFECTS:
    - Hematological (neutropenia, lymphopenia, anemia, thrombocytopenia), astenia, nausea, vomiting, visual symptoms, infection.

Satraplatin

[Sternberg CN, *Oncology* **68**(1): 2–9, 2005]

- A novel oral platinum complex with activity in cisplatin-resistant human tumor lines.

- Randomized, phase III trial of prednisone ± satraplatin in 50 patients.
  - RESULTS:
    - Favoring combination with satraplatin.
    - Median overall survival → 14.9 vs 11.9 months.
    - > 50% PSA response → 33% vs 8.7%.
    - Progression-free survival → 5.2 vs 2.5 months.
  - SIDE-EFFECTS:
    - Neutropenia (15%).
    - Thrombocytopenia (30%).
    - Diarrhea (7%).
    - Vomiting (7%).

Calcitriol (DN-101)

[Beer TM, *Cancer* **97**: 1217–1224, 2003]

[Beer TM, *J Clin Oncol* **21**: 123–128, 2003]
[Beer TM, *Proc Am Soc Clin Oncol* **24**: 382, 2005]

- Biologically active metabolite of vitamin D.

- Several mechanisms of action.
  - Inhibition of proliferation, resulting in cell-cycle arrest.
  - Differentiation.
  - Induction of apoptosis.

- Single agent, weekly calcitriol in hormone-naive patients appeared to have anti-tumor activity in an uncontrolled study.

- Phase II study of weekly calcitriol in addition to docetaxel in 37 chemotherapy-naive patients with HRPC.
  - RESULTS:
    - > 50% PSA ↓ in 81% of patients.
    - Median time to progression → 11.4 months.
    - Median survival → 19.5 months.

- A randomized, placebo-controlled trial of docetaxel ± calcitriol in 250 chemotherapy-naive patients with HRPC.
  - RESULTS:
    - Favored calcitriol over placebo.
    - PSA response: 58% vs 49%, primary endpoint.
    - Tumor response: 28% vs 20%.
    - Median survival: 23.5 vs 16.4 months, secondary endpoint.

Growth factor receptor antagonists

Epidermal growth factor receptor

[Slovin SF, *Proc Am Soc Clin Oncol* **16**: 311a, 1997]
[Rosenthal M, *Proc Am Soc Clin Oncol* **22**: 416, 2003]

- Cetuximab is an anti-epitheloid growth factor receptor (anti-EGFR) monoclonal antibody that prevents activation of receptor tyrosine kinase; it is approved for treatment of colon cancer.
  - Combination of cetuximab with doxorubicin in 18 patients with HRPC showed stabilization of PSA for a median of 4 months in 28% of patients.

- Gefitinib is an oral EGFR tyrosine kinase inhibitor, used in the treatment of non-small cell lung cancer.
  - In a phase II trial of gefitinib in HRPC, PSA responses were infrequent and many patients were found to have early progression.

HER-2

[Chee KG, *Proc Am Soc Clin Oncol* **22**: 403 (abstract 1620), 2003]
[Morris MJ, *Cancer* **94**: 980–986, 2002]

- Trastuzumab is a humanized monoclonal antibody that targets the extracellular domain of *HER-2*, and has significant activity in *HER-2* expressing breast cancer.

- Results on *HER-2* expression in prostate cancer, as determined by immunohistochemistry, vary widely.
  - In a phase II trial in patients with advanced prostate cancer, trastuzumab alone produced no responses in 23 patients with either *HER-2* (–) or *HER-2* (+) disease.
  - Another phase II trial of trastuzumab and docetaxel in HRPC was closed early due to lack of response.

Platelet-derived growth factor receptor

[Rao KV, *Proc Am Soc Clin Oncol* **22**: 409 (abstract 1645), 2003]

- Imatinib (Gleevac) is a specific inhibitor of the BCR-ABL, c-kit, and platelet-derived growth factor (PDGF) receptor tyrosine kinases.
  - A phase II trial of imatinib as a single agent in 17 patients with hormone-naive progressive prostate cancer after local therapy demonstrated stable disease in 6 (35%) patients.

Anti-angiogenetic agents

Thalidomide

[Figg WD, *Clin Cancer Res* **7**: 1888–1893, 2001]
[Drake MJ, *Br J Cancer* **88**: 822–827, 2003]
[Dahut WL, *J Clin Oncol* **22**: 2532–2539, 2004)

- A sedative, anti-inflammatory, and immunosuppressive agent.

- Blocks activity of bFGF, VEGF, and interkeukin-6.

- A phase II, clinical trial randomized 63 patients with chemotherapy-naive HRPC to a low-dose group (200 mg/day, 50 patients) or a high-dose group (dose escalation up to 1200 mg, 13 patients).
  - The high-dose group was terminated early due to a lack of efficacy and poor tolerance.

- 9 (15%) patients in the low-dose group showed a PSA decline of > 50%.

- Another phase II study of low-dose thalidomide in 20 patients with HRPC showed a 50% PSA decline in 3 (15%) ♂.

- Combination with docetaxel in a randomized, phase II trial of 53 patients with chemotherapy-naive HRPC resulted in a > 50% PSA ↓ in 53% of patients, compared with 35% for docetaxel alone.
  - Progression-free survival and overall survival at 18 months were improved with combination therapy (5.9 vs 3.7 months and 68% vs 43%, respectively).
  - SIDE-EFFECTS:
    - Thromboembolic events, constipation, depression, confusion, dry eye, dry mouth, myalgias/arthralgias.

Bevacizumab (Avastin)

[Picus J, *Proc Am Soc Clin Oncol* **22**: 393 (abstract 1578), 2003]

- Recombinant, humanized anti-VEGF murine monoclonal antibody.

- In an ongoing, phase II trial of bevacizumab, docetaxel, and estramustine in 79 patients with chemotherapy-naive HRPC.
  - RESULTS:
    - 65% of patients have shown > 50% PSA ↓.
    - 53% with measurable disease have had a partial response.

Proapoptotic agents

Bcl-2 antisense (oblimersen)

[Chi KN, *Proc Am Soc Clin Oncol* **22**: 393, 2003]

- Bcl-2 is a mitochondrial-associated protein conferring resistance to apoptosis.

- It is overexpressed in prostate cancer.

- Oblimersen (G3139) is an antisense oligonucleotide directed to the first six codons of the initiating sequence of the human bcl-2 mRNA.

- A phase II study of oblimersen in combination with docetaxel in 31 ♂ with metastatic HRPC yielded a > 50% PSA ↓ in 15 (48%) patients and a partial response in 27% of patients.
  - 42% of patients experienced grade 3–4 neutropenia.

Other novel targeted agents

Bortezomib (Velcade)

[Dreicer R, *Proc Am Soc Clin Oncol* **23**: 418 (abstract 4654), 2004]

- Boronic acid dipeptide that inhibits 26S proteasome activity.
- A phase I trial with 48 patients demonstrated a response rate of 11%.
- A phase I/II trial of bortezomib with docetaxel in 100 patients with metastatic HRPC.
  - RESULTS:
    - > 50% of PSA $\downarrow$ in 24% of patients.
  - SIDE-EFFECTS:
    - Diarrhea, nausea, fatigue, constipation, peripheral neuropathy, anorexia.

Atrasentan

[Carducci M, *Proc Am Soc Clin Oncol* **23**: 383, 2004]
[Vogelzang NJ, *Proc Am Soc Clin Oncol* **24**: abstract 269, 2005]

- Highly selective oral endothelin receptor antagonist.
- Endothelin-1 is a potent vasoconstrictor produced by prostate cancer and appears to have a role in prostate cancer progression and morbidity.
- In a phase III, placebo-controlled trial of 809 patients with metastatic prostate cancer, atrasentan therapy was associated with smaller increases in serum PSA (183 vs 137 days) and markers of bone turnover, as well as a modest delay in time to clinical progression (155 vs 71 days).
- A meta-analysis of two randomized, placebo-controlled clinical trials of 1,002 patients with HRPC showed a statistically significant delay in time to disease progression (14%), time to bone pain (18%), time to PSA progression (22%), and time to bone alkaline phosphatase progression (46%) for atrasentan 10 mg p.o.
  - SIDE-EFFECTS:
    - Headache, peripheral edema, rhinitis.

Immunotherapeutic agents

Granulocyte-macrophage colony-stimulating factor (GM-CSF)

[Dreicer R, *Invest New Drugs* **19**: 261–264, 2001]

- Supposed to ↑ the efficiency of tumor antigen presentation and subsequent activation of tumor-specific cytotoxic T-lymphocytes.

- 16 patients treated with GM-CSF 250 µg s.c. 3 times weekly.
  - 6 demonstrated a 10–15% ↓ in PSA levels for up to 6 months.

GVAX

[Small E, *Proc Am Soc Clin Oncol* **23**: 396 (abstract 4565), 2004]
[Small E, *Proc Am Soc Clin Oncol* **24**(1): 141 (abstract 280), 2005]

- Cancer vaccines of tumor cells that have been genetically modified to secrete GM-CSF.

- Phase II trial results in 80 patients with HRPC 32% showed a modest PSA ↓, and 62% had stable or improved markers of bone turnover.

Provenge (APC8015)

[Small EJ, *Proc Am Soc Clin Oncol* **4**: abstract 4500, 2005]

- An immunotherapeutic product consisting of autologous dendritic cells loaded ex vivo with a recombinant fusion protein of prostatic acid phosphatase linked to GM-CSF, designed to initiate a T-cell mediated immune response against prostatic acid phosphatase, which is overexpressed in 95% of prostate cancer cells.

- A randomized, phase II study in 127 chemotherapy-naive patients with HRPC and a Gleason score < 8 found improved progression-free survival and overall survival (25.9 vs 22.0 months).
  - SIDE-EFFECTS:
    - Grade 1–2 infusion-related fevers and rigors.

Vaccinia virus/fowlpox virus

[Kaufman HL, *J Clin Oncol* **22**: 2122–2132, 2004]
[Gulley J, *Proc 2005 Multidisc Prostate Cancer Symp*, abstract 287]

- Viral vectors mimic natural infection and induce potent immune responses.

- Prime/boost vaccine strategy using vaccinia and fowlpox virus expressing human PSA to induce T-cell responses directed against PSA.

- In a randomized, phase II trial of 64 patients with PSA progression after definitive local therapy, 45% of patients remained free of PSA progression at 19 months.

- Another phase II trial of 32 chemotherapy-naive patients with metastatic HRPC and progressive disease randomized patients into four groups: vaccine alone, vaccine with GM-CSF, or vaccine with two different doses of fowlpox GM-CSF.
  - 5/16 patients had PSA declines during a period of 3 months.
  - One partial response at 8 months with > 50% decline in hilar adenopathy.
  - One patient with stable disease at 9 months.
- Well-tolerated.

Anti prostate-specific membrane antigen J591 monoclonal antibody

[Milowsky MI, *J Clin Oncol* **22**: 2522–2531, 2004]

- Prostate-specific membrane antigen (PSMA) is a cell-surface glycoprotein expressed in both benign and malignant prostate tissue.
- J591 binds the extracellular PSMA epitope.
- Yttrium-90 labeled J591 demonstrated significant anti-tumor activity in 2/29 patients with advanced androgen-independent prostate cancer.
- Dose-limiting toxicities: thrombocytopenia, bleeding.

24

Complications of radical prostatectomy

[Brown JA, *Urol Oncol* **22**: 102–106, 2004]
[Menon M, *Urol Clin North Am* **31**: 701–718, 2004]

- Since the use of serum prostatic-specific antigen, early detection of prostate cancer has ↑ significantly, resulting in more radical prostatectomies.

- Radical prostatectomy can be performed by one of several methods.
  - Perineal.
  - Retropubic.
  - Laparoscopic.
  - Robotic.

- Initially, radical prostatectomy was performed by the perineal approach, as described by Kuchler in 1868 and popularized by Young in 1905.
  - This became the procedure of choice for radical prostatectomy until recognition of the value of a pelvic lymphadenectomy in the 1970s, at which time the retropubic approach replaced the perineal approach.

- Laparoscopic radical prostatectomy was first performed by Schuessler in 1997 and robotic radical prostatectomy, using the Da Vinci surgical robot, was first performed by Binder in 2000.
  - Although minimally invasive techniques are feasible with equivalent short-term results to those of conventional radical prostatectomy, we still await long-term results, including oncological outcomes, to determine their efficacy.

- Mortality statistics from radical prostatectomy were compiled from Medicare claims.

- 30-day mortality rate, 0.5%; 1-year mortality rate, 1.8%.
  [Mark DH, *J Urol* **152**: 896–898, 1994]

• Morbidity rates have been stratified by age.
  A 4% complication rate was noted in ♂ in their forties, 9% in those
  in their fifties, 11% in those in their sixties, and 14% in those in
  their seventies.
  [Catalona WJ, *Geriatrics* **54**: 49–54, 1999]

• Morbidity following radical prostatectomy depends on several factors:
  – Patient medical comorbidities.
  – Prior surgeries.
  – Prior radiation.
  – Prostate size.
  – Patient anatomy.
  – Volume of prostate cancer.
  – Use of preoperative hormone ablation.
  – Surgeon experience.
  – Other factors.

• Complications can be divided into two types.
  • Perioperative (at the time of surgery or within 30 days of surgery).
    – Hemorrhage.
    – Rectal injury.
    – Oliguria/anuria.
    – Lymphocele.
    – Nerve injury.
    – Cardiovascular.
    – Infection.
    – Foley catheter loss.
    – Perineal pain syndrome.
  • Postoperative (> 30 days).
    – Bladder neck contracture.
    – Incontinence.
    – Impotence.

Hemorrhage

[Davies BJ, *J Urol* **64**: 712–716, 2004]
[Haab F, *Br J Urol* **74**: 626–629, 1994]
[Hoznek A, *Curr Opin Urol* **15**: 173–180, 2005]
[Kaufman JD, *Urology* **66**: 561–563, 2005]
[Leandri P, *J Urol* **147**: 883–887, 1992]

[Salonia A, *Urology* **64**: 95–100, 2004]
[Schostak M, *BJU Intl* **96**: 316–319, 2005]
[Weldon VE, *J Urol* **158**: 1470–1475, 1997]

- Blood loss reports from radical prostatectomy have been highly variable.
  - Generally, the open technique has been associated with a greater degree of blood loss than the perineal, laparoscopic, or robotic techniques.

- Common sites of hemorrhage.
  - Dorsal venous complex.
    - Most common source of bleeding.
    - Incising the endopelvic fascia laterally and distally may decrease bleeding from the dorsal venous complex before dividing.
    - If troublesome bleeding is encountered from the dorsal venous complex, it may be completely divided and oversewn.
    - Blood loss has been shown to decrease with increased surgeon experience.
  - Hypogastric vein.
    - Can be injured performing pelvic lymph node dissection or during trocar placement.
  - Arterial branches to the prostate and seminal vesicles.
    - Can be controlled by clips (nerve-sparing) or cautery (non-nerve-sparing).
    - Troublesome with any technique.
  - Bulb of the penis.
    - Seen in the perineal approach when dissection proceeds too far anteriorly when trying to divide the rectourethralis.

- Delayed bleeding.
  - Conservative treatment is recommended for hemodynamically stable patients.
  - Reoperation, indicated for major bleeding and hemodynamic instability, may facilitate both healing of the vesicourethral anastomosis and removal of the urinary catheter.
  - Continence also appears to be better preserved if the hematoma is evacuated.

- Recent studies have shown decreased blood loss with spinal anesthesia compared to general anesthesia in patients undergoing radical retropubic prostatectomy.

- Delayed intraoperative hydration, or limiting intravenous fluids before completion of dissection of the prostate, appears to reduce blood loss during radical retropubic prostatectomy.

- One group recently proposed a new method of reducing blood loss in patients undergoing radical retropubic prostatectomy.
  - The new method comprised reducing the intravenously applied volume, using an epidural catheter, and maintaining a 25–30° Trendelenburg position.

Rectal injury

[Brehmer B, *Eur Urol* **40**: 139–143, 2001]
[Harpster LE, *J Urol* **154**: 1435, 1995]
[Katz R, *Urology* **62**: 310–313, 2003]
[Lassen PM, *Urology* **45**: 266–269, 1995]
[Lepor H, *J Urol* **166**: 1729–1733, 2001]
[McLaren RH, *Urology* **42**: 401–405, 1993]
[Walsh P, *J Urol* **147**: 905–907, 1992]

- Incidence is 0–3.6% of patients undergoing radical prostatectomy.

- Can occur with any technique, although the incidence has been shown to be higher with the perineal approach. Rectal injury in this series, however, was still only 1–2% with the perineal approach.

- Preoperative rectal preparation with enema is recommended. It has been shown that rectal injury after bowel preparation is associated with a lower risk of complications, including rectourinary fistula and abscess formation.

- Risk factors.
  - Previous radiation.
  - Rectal surgery.
  - Periprostatic inflammation due to previous transurethral resection or recent biopsy.

- Injury often occurs during apical dissection of the prostate and division of the rectourethralis muscle.

- Acceptable to repair primarily.
  - Debride devitalized tissue.
  - Repair with a two-layer closure of the mucosal and muscular layer.
  - Interpose the omental flap between the rectal repair and the vesicourethral anastomosis by creating a small opening in the retroperitoneum.
  - Perform anal dilatation.
  - Alternatives include a pedicalized flap of peritoneum or perirectal fat.

- Large injuries or gross soiling can be treated with a diverting colostomy.
- Similar closure has been reported using laparoscopy, with excellent success.

Oliguria/anuria

[Catalona WJ, *J Urol* **162**: 433–438, 1999]
[Crisci A, *Urology* **62**: 941, 2003]
[Hammerer, *Urologe A* **34**: 334–342, 1995]
[Hautmann, *Urology* **43**: 47–51, 1994]
[Leandri P, *J Urol* **147**: 883–887, 1992]
[Walsh PC, *Campbell's Urology*, 7th edn. WB Saunders, Philadelphia, PA, 1998]

- Ureteral injury.
  - Incidence is 0.05 → 1.6% of cases.
  - Can occur with any technique.
  - Sites of injury.
    - Division of bladder neck.
      - Injury can occur, especially if there is benign prostatic hypertrophy and J-hooking of the ureters.
      - Administer intravenous indigo carmine to identify ureteral orifices.
    - Posterior dissection of the seminal vesicles.
      - Ureters run anterolateral to the seminal vesicles and cross toward the midline above the trigone.
      - Avoid blind placement of sutures in this area.
      - Cannulate the ureter with feeding tubes or perform a retrograde pyelogram if injury suspected.
  - Perform a ureteroneocystotomy if injury is recognized.

- Anastomotic leak.
  - Incidence varies in the range 0–22.3%. Most series report 1–2%.
  - Directly related to the quality of the anastomosis.
  - Anastomotic leaks usually resolve with adequate drainage.
  - Re-exploration is discouraged, as the tissues are friable.
  - Fever or pelvic pain may indicate an undrained pelvic fluid collection; this can often be drained percutaneously.
  - Complete urethrovesical anastomotic disruption is rare and is often a result of hematoma or seroma. Healing should occur with the catheter acting as a stent. Bladder neck contractures are common in this clinical scenario.

- Acute tubular necrosis.
  - Ensure that the patient is adequately hydrated.
  - It is important to rule out other etiologies of renal dysfunction.

- Foley obstruction.
  - Can usually be treated with gentle irrigation.

- Trigonal edema.
  - Often a diagnosis of exclusion.

Lymphocele

[Gill IS, *J Urol* **153**: 706–711, 1995]
[Gilliland JD, *Radiology* **171**: 227–229, 1989]
[Pepper RJ, *BJU Intl* **95**: 772–775, 2005]
[Rassweiler J, *J Urol* **169**: 1689–1693, 2003]
[Sibert L, *Ann Urol* **28**: 202–206, 1994]
[Sommerkamp H, *Eur Urol* **12**: 265–269, 1986]

- The incidence of symptomatic lymphoceles is 4.7–14.8% after pelvic lymph node dissection during open radical retropubic prostatectomy.
  - The incidence appears to decrease with laparoscopic pelvic lymph node dissection or limited node dissections.

- The incidence of subclinical lymphoceles is 40%.

- Most lymphoceles remain asymptomatic and resolve spontaneously.

- Risk factors.
  - Pelvic lymph node dissection.
  - Surgical technique.
  - Tumor-bearing nodes.

- Symptomatic lymphoceles may present with abdominal pain, lower extremity swelling, scrotal edema, and fever if infected.
  - Treatment is percutaneous drainage under computerized tomography or ultrasonography guidance.
  - If drainage persists, sclerotherapy and laparoscopic peritoneal marsupialization with or without omentopexy is associated with success rates of > 90%.

Nerve injury

[Ahearn GS, *South Med J* **92**: 809–811, 1999]
[Burnett AL, *J Urol* **151**: 163–165, 1994]
[Kavoussi LR, *J Urol* **149**: 322–325, 1993]

- The incidence is 0.5–1% (similar with all techniques).

- Obturator nerve injury.
  - A rare complication of pelvic lymphadenectomy after transection, excessive electrocoagulation, or compression secondary to retractors.
  - Also seen in perineal, laparoscopic, and robotic techniques secondary to patient positioning.
  - Greatest risk of transection is during proximal dissection of the node packet, in which the nerve may sometimes course upward into the packet.
  - Injury weakens thigh abduction, with diminished sensation on the medial aspect of the thigh.
  - Most cases resolve spontaneously. Transection may be repaired primarily.

- Femoral nerve injury.
  - A well-recognized complication due to retractor injury on the psoas muscle.
  - Injury results in quadriceps weakness and paresthesia of the anteromedial aspect of the thigh.

Cardiovascular effects

[ACC/AHA, *Circulation* **93**: 1278–1317, 1996]
[Goldman L, *New Engl J Med* **297**: 845–850, 1997]
[Lepor H, *J Urol* **166**: 1729–1733, 2001]
[Lerner SE, *Oncology* **9**: 379–382, 1995]
[Sieber PR, *J Urol* **158**: 869–871, 1997]

- Pulmonary embolus/deep venous thrombosis.
  - The incidence varies in the range 0.5–3%.
  - It is the most common cause of operative and perioperative mortality in patients undergoing radical prostatectomy.
  - Preventive measures, such as sequential devices and anticoagulation in the form of low molecular or subcutaneous heparin, are commonly used, although data demonstrating benefit are conflicting.
  - Early ambulation, on the same day as surgery, is considered important.
  - Any patient presenting with unexplained fever, leg swelling, or leg tenderness should be evaluated using Doppler ultrasonography of the lower extremity.

- Myocardial infarction.
  - The incidence is rare but significant.

- Key to avoiding cardiac complications is preoperative risk assessment.
- Clinical predictors of increased perioperative cardiac risk (major).
  - Unstable coronary syndrome.
  - Decompensated congestive heart failure.
  - Significant arrhythmias.
- Preventive measures.
  - Aggressive treatment of hypertension.
  - Avoidance of hypovolemia.
  - Maintenance of hematocrit > 30%.

Infection

[Catalona WJ, *J Urol* **162**: 433–438, 1999]
[Lerner SE, *Oncology* **9**: 379–882, 1995]

- The incidence varies in the range 1–3%.

- Prophylactic antibiotics.
  - Preoperative antibiotics should be directed towards skin flora.
  - We use a first-generation cephalosporin preoperatively, which is continued for 24 hours.
  - Preoperative urine culture is advisable to identify infection.
  - All infections must be treated prior to surgery.

- Wound infection.
  - The most common type of infection in the postoperative period.
  - Risk factors.
    - Urinary extravasation.
    - Bleeding.
    - Excessive subcutaneous fat.
  - Early, aggressive treatment is recommended.
  - Urine leak or abscess should be suspected for prolonged drainage.

- Urinary tract infection.
  - Increased risk with an indwelling catheter.
  - Prolonged antibiotic prophylaxis following surgery is controversial, and benefit has not been clearly demonstrated.

Foley catheter loss

[Guillonneau B, *Prostate* **39**: 71–75, 1999]
[Palmer J, *Urology* **47**: 23–28, 1996]
[Tiguert R, *Urology* **63**: 513–517, 2004]

- The incidence is rare but significant.
- Guidelines for Foley catheter loss.
  - < 5 days postoperatively.
    - Perform a cystoscopy for Foley placement over the guide wire. Some advocate attempting gentle Foley catheter replacement prior to cystoscopy. If there is any concern regarding placement, cystoscopy can be performed.
    - If it is not possible to place the catheter by cystoscopy, place a suprapubic cystotomy tube and attempt antegrade passage of a guidewire and retrograde passage of a urethral catheter.
    - Suprapubic cystotomy is also recommended during this time period if clot retention or severe hematuria develops. Catheter exchange is discouraged.
    - If it is not possible to place any catheter, reoperation may be required.
  - > 5 days postoperatively.
    - Consider leaving the Foley catheter out as long as the patient has not developed urinary retention.
    - Gentle passage of a catheter is possible at this stage, if needed.

Perineal pain syndrome

[Arai Y, *Int J Urol* **10**: 430–434, 2003]
[Melman A, *J Urol* **171**: 786–790, 2004]
[McCanse W, Presented at AUA SCS Annual Meeting, abstract 23, 2005]
[Palou J, *Scand J Urol Nephrol* **31**: 493–495, 1997]
[Weizer AZ, *Urology* **62**: 693–697, 2003]

- The incidence is obviously highest in the perineal approach, but overall narcotic use is low.
- Interestingly, it has been reported after laparoscopic and robotic techniques.
  - Laparoscopic series reported an incidence in 4.7% of cases.
  - Robotic series reported an incidence in 7.5% of cases.
- One case of perineal pain following open radical retropubic prostatectomy was attributed to a metal clip protruding into the urethra through the urethrovesical anastomosis.
- The etiology is unknown.
  - Temporary neural or muscular dysfunction may play a role.

Bladder neck contracture

[Besarani D, *BJU Intl* **94**: 1245–1247, 2004]
[Kastakopoulos A, *Urol Intl* **72**: 17–20, 2004]
[Surya BV, *J Urol* **143**: 755–758, 1990]

- The incidence is 0.5–17% following radical prostatectomy (5–10% in most series).

- The incidence is lowest with the perineal, laparoscopic, and robotic techniques.

- Risk factors.
  - Urine extravasation.
  - Poor mucosal approximation.
  - Pelvic hematoma.
  - Suture reaction (use absorbable monofilament).
  - Ischemia (excessive thinning or mobilization of the bladder neck).

- If possible, place posterior urethral sutures before division of the posterior urethra and rectourethralis (the mucosa retracts posteriorly, resulting in urethral thinning).

- Presenting symptoms range from ↓ urinary stream to urinary incontinence.

- Cold knife incision or dilatation is preferred due to the risk of urinary incontinence after electrosurgical resection.

Incontinence

[Bianco FJ, *Urology* **66**: 83–94, 2005]
[Catalona WJ, *J Urol* **162**: 433–438, 1999]
[Eastham JA, *J Urol* **156**: 1707–1713, 1996]
[Fenelye MR, *Lancet* **353**: 2091, 1999]
[House JC, Presented at AUA Meeting, abstract 1007, 2005]
[Shekarriz B, *Urol Clin North Am* **28**: 639–653, 2001]
[Slabaugh TK, *J Urol* **172**: 2545–2548, 2004]
[Stanford JL, *JAMA* **283**: 354–360, 2000]
[Weldon VE, *J Urol* **158**: 1470–1475, 1997]

- Most patients are incontinent after initial catheter removal.

- A wide range of incidence has been reported due to the lack of a universal definition of incontinence.

- Incontinence can generally be subclassified into complete or severe incontinence and stress incontinence.

- The reported incidences of complete incontinence vary in the range 0–17% and that of stress incontinence in the range 0–35%.

- The Prostate Cancer Outcomes Study encompassed six geographical regions and found 14% of patients to have frequent urinary leakage or no urinary control at 5 years after open radical prostatectomy. This was increased from 10% at 2 years.

- Perineal radical prostatectomy incontinence rates have been reported to be around 5%, perhaps due to better visualization and direct mucosal-to-mucosal anastomosis.

- Rates of incontinence with laparoscopic and robotic techniques are comparable to those with the open technique.

- Risk factors.
  - Surgical technique.
  - Patient age.
  - Neurovascular bundle resection (conflicting).
  - Anastomotic stricture.

- Incontinence is generally secondary to intrinsic sphincter deficiency, although bladder instability may contribute in some cases. Urodynamics is useful when planning intervention.

- Kegel exercises and biofeedback are excellent first-line treatment options.

- Anticholinergics, α-agonists, periurethral collagen injections, slings, and artificial urinary sphincter are options available for long-term and bothersome urinary incontinence.

Impotence

[Catalona WJ, J Urol **162**: 433–438, 1999]
[Cooperberg MR, Urology **61**: 190–196, 2003]
[Mulhall JP, Int J Impot Res **8**: 91–94, 1996]
[Rabbani F, J Urol **171**(Suppl): 310–311, 2004]
[Slabaugh TK, J Urol **172**: 2545–2548, 2004]
[Stanford JL, JAMA **283**: 354–360, 2000]
[Walsh PC, J Urol **128**: 492–497, 1982]
[Weldon VE, J Urol **158**: 1470, 1997]

- The incidence is similar to incontinence rates following radical prostatectomy. A wide range of incidence of impotence has been reported due to the lack of a universal method of measuring sexual function.

- Postoperative potency rates reported in the literature vary in the range 3–97%. Potency is generally defined as the ability to achieve an erection suitable for intercourse or an International Index of Erectile Function (IIEF) score of > 15.

- It is the consensus of most urologists that impotence rates after radical prostatectomy have ↓ since the adoption of Walsh and Donker's nerve-sparing technique.

- The incidence of impotence in two recent large series was reported as 32%.
    - The Prostate Cancer Outcomes Study group found that 28% of ♂ were impotent at 5 years vs 22% at 2 years following open surgery.

- ~ 60% of all prostatectomy patients report significant emotional distress related to their sexual dysfunction.

- Impotence rates after perineal radical prostatectomy have been reported to be around 30%.

- Rates of impotence with laparoscopic and robotic techniques are comparable to those with the open technique.

- ↑ potency rates in robotic prostatectomy patients may be obtained using a prostatic-fascia-sparing technique in addition to conventional nerve sparing.
[Menon M, J Urol **174**: 2291–2295, 2005]

- Risk factors.
    - Age.
    - Clinical and pathological stage.
    - Surgical technique (extent of nerve sparing).

- Recovery of sexual function may continue for up to 4 years following surgery.

- The etiology of impotence after radical prostatectomy is multifactorial.

- Phosphodiesterase inhibitors have been successful in treating postoperative radical prostatectomy impotence.
    - Sildenafil citrate has been shown to restore sexual function in 80% of patients who are unable to have intercourse 12 months or more after surgery.

- Other treatment options for motivated patients include intraurethal suppository, intercavernosal injection, vacuum assist device, and penile prosthesis.

CHAPTER 25

Side-effects of treatment

Prostatectomy

Urinary toxicity

[Stanford JL, JAMA **283**: 354–360, 2000]

- Complications are variable and have been found to be dependent on the experience of the surgeon.
  [Begg CB, N Engl J Med **356**: 1138–1144, 2002]

- Immediate postoperative complications include pelvic pain and incontinence.

- Incontinence is almost universal immediately after radical prostatectomy (RP), and lasts for several weeks.

- The incidence of postoperative stress incontinence is 5–57%.

- 20–35% of patients will require pads for protection for > 1 year following RP.

- 5–10% of patients will require long-term use of diapers following RP.

- The level of urinary control following RP at 24 months is age dependent.
  - 27% and 14% of ♂ aged 75–79 years had no urinary control or frequent leakage, respectively, compared with 5% and 1% of ♂ aged < 60 years.

Erectile dysfunction

[Stanford JL, JAMA **283**: 354–360, 2000]
[Talcott JA, J Natl Cancer Inst **89**: 1117–1123, 1997]
[Teloken C, Cancer Control **8**: 540–545, 2001]

- The incidence of impotence following retropubic RP ranges between 35% and 100%.

- Predictors of sexual function after RP include baseline sexual function, age, type of surgery, and race.

- Sexual function quality-of-life scores immediately post-treatment and at 1 year are significantly worse for those patients who have undergone RP (10.3 and 21.6) than for those who have received radiation therapy (34.4 and 34.1) for prostate cancer.
  [Lubeck D, Urology **58**(Suppl 2A): 94–100, 2001]

- Sexual function improves to some degree within 2 years following surgery.
  The proportion of ♂ without erections firm enough for intercourse has been shown to decrease from 80% at 6 months following RP to 60% at 24 months.
  – In addition, the proportion of ♂ who had no difficulties maintaining an erection at 6 months following surgery was 2%, vs 7% at 24 months.

- Nerve-sparing RPs have better potency rates postoperatively compared with non-nerve-sparing RP.

- The proportions of patients who were able to have erections firm enough for intercourse at 24 months following non-nerve-sparing, unilateral nerve-sparing, and bilateral nerve-sparing surgery were 34%, 41%, and 44%, respectively.

- A non-retrospective cohort study has challenged the idea that nerve-sparing RPs improve postoperative sexual function compared to non-nerve-sparing RPs.
  – It was found that ♂ with preoperative impotence and more advanced cancers receive nerve-sparing procedures less often.
  – Previous benefit of nerve-sparing surgery may be the result of patient selection and not technique.

- Older patients treated with RP have a higher incidence of impotence.
  – In patients aged < 60 years → 39% had erections firm enough for intercourse vs 19% of patients aged 75–79 years.

- Sexual function post-RP varies by race.
  - 38.4% of black ♂.
  - 25.9% of Hispanic ♂.
  - 21.3% of white ♂ reported firm erections at 24 months.

External beam radiation

- There are several critical organs located around the prostate that are subject to side-effects secondary to radiation.

- The likelihood and severity of side-effects is directly related to the total dose of radiation the organs receive and the volume of the organ that receives that dose.

- With the introduction of three-dimensional conformal radiation therapy (3D-CRT) and intensity-modulated radiation therapy (IMRT), radiation oncologists are able to decrease doses to critical structures while escalating the radiation dose to the prostate.

- Estimates of complication rates have improved considerably as a result of these newer dose volume, histogram-based therapies; this is not reflected in older data.

Rectal toxicity

[Denton AS, *Br J Cancer* **87**: 134–143, 2002]

- Possible acute rectal side-effects include increased bowel movement frequency, pain on defecation, hematochezia, rectal incontinence, and rectal spasm.

- Rare late complications include rectal bleeding, ulceration, perforation, and/or fistula formation.

- Patients with previous bowel surgery, T_4 tumors, or inflammatory bowel disease have an increased risk of rectal ulceration or fistula.

- The risks for the late complications of proctitis, rectal stricture, or rectal ulceration are 10%, 5%, and 2%, respectively, in ♂ treated with traditional pelvic fields.
  [Pilepich, *Int J Radiat Oncol Biol Phys* **13**: 1007–1012, 1987]

- The incidence of rectal bleeding ↑ from 12% to 20% when receiving radiation doses > 70 Gy with non-3D-CRT techniques.

- Patients undergoing dose escalation with 3D-CRT have higher rates of gastrointestinal toxicities than those treated with conventional fields to lower doses.
  [Pollack MD, *Int J Radiat Oncol Biol Phys* **53**: 1097–1105, 2002]

- When evaluating plans for 3D-CRT with dose volume histograms an ↑ in late rectal toxicity was found when > 25% of rectum received ≥ 70 Gy (37% vs 13%).
  [Storey MR, *Int J Radiat Oncol Biol Phys* **48**: 635–642, 2000]

- In patients undergoing 3D-CRT it was found that 118 (86%) had no acute gastrointestinal toxicity, with only 14% requiring medication for relief (grade 2).
  - 157 (94%) had no late rectal toxicity, with 6% developing late grade 2 (rectal bleeding). There were no grade 3 or higher toxicities.
    [Zelefsky MJ, *J Clin Oncol* **17**: 517–522, 1999]

- Evaluation of high-dose IMRT has shown superior rates of rectal toxicities compared with conventional fields and 3D-CRT.
  - Actuarial acute and late toxicities were 4.5% and 4%, respectively.
  - No patients experienced grade 3 or higher acute toxicity, and the rate of late grade 3 toxicity was 0.1%, with no late grade 4 or 5 toxicities.
    [Zelefsky MJ, *Int J Radiat Oncol Biol Phys* **53**: 1111–1116, 2002]

- A prospective randomized trial evaluating oral sulfasalazine + rectal steroids vs rectal sulcrafate for radiation proctitis found superior clinical improvement with sulcrafate (odds ratio 14) but no difference on endoscopic evaluation.
  [Kochhar R, *Dig Dis Sci* **36**: 103–107, 1999]

- The use of metronidazole with mesalazine, and betamethasone enema was found to be superior to the use of mesalazine and betamethasone alone for radiation-induced proctitis.
  - The incidence of rectal bleeding and mucosal ulcers were significantly lower in the metronidazole group at 4 weeks, 3 months, and 1 year, both clinically and endoscopically.
    [Cavcic J, *Croat Med J* **41**: 314–318, 2000]

- A prospective randomized trial showed no benefit using short-chain fatty acids to treat radiation-induced proctitis.
  [Talley NA, *Dis Colon Rectum* **40**: 1046–1050, 1997]

- Thermal coagulation therapy has been shown to have a statistical benefit in controlling radiation-induced rectal bleeding.
  [Jensen DM, *Gastrointest Endosc* **45**: 20–25, 1997]

- Hyperbaric oxygen is thought to have some benefit in treating refractory chronic radiation-induced large bowel injury; however, there is little evidence to support this.
  [Denton AS, *Br J Cancer* **87**: 134–143, 2002]

Urinary toxicity

- Acute bladder side-effects include increased urinary frequency, increased nocturia, urgency, hematuria, dysuria, bladder spasms, and urinary incontinence.

- Late complication may involve hemorrhagic cystitis or ulceration, bladder contracture, and incontinence.

- 50% of patients have significant prostate shrinkage in response to radiation therapy.
  - This shrinkage is usually not associated with any urinary symptoms, although it is possible to see either improvement or worsening of urinary function.

- Strictures of the urethra are uncommon and occur most frequently in those patients that have previously undergone transurethral resection of the prostate (TURP).
  [Seymore CH, *Int J Radiat Oncol Biol Phys* **12**: 1596–1600, 1986]
  [Sandhu AS, *Int J Radiat Oncol Biol Phys* **48**: 643–647, 2000]

- In patients receiving whole-pelvis irradiation + 3 years of androgen-deprivation therapy (ADT) there is a statistical ↑ in grade 1–3 urinary incontinence (29% vs 16%) vs patients who received whole-pelvis radiation therapy alone.
  [Bolla M, *N Engl J Med* **337**: 295–300, 1997]

- Escalating the prostate dose to 78 Gy using 3D-CRT after the initial pelvic field does not lead to ↑ acute or late urinary toxicities when compared with patients treated with conventional fields to 70 Gy.
  [Storey MR, *Int J Radiat Oncol Biol Phys* **48**: 635–642, 2000]

- Among 137 ♂ undergoing 3D-CRT.
  [Zelefsky MJ, *J Clin Oncol* **17**: 517–522, 1999]
  - 58% had no or mild (grade 1) acute urinary symptoms; 42% required medication for relief of symptoms (grade 2).
  - There was no incidence of acute urinary retention.
  - No late grade 2 urinary toxicity was observed in 91% of patients.
  - Late grade 3 toxicity (urethral stricture) occurred in 2 (1%) patients.

Erectile dysfunction

- Impotence after conventional external beam radiation therapy (EBRT) is not an uncommon complication.
  [Banker FL, *Int J Radiat Oncol Biol Phys* **15**: 219–220, 1988]
  - Incidence rates range from 22% to 50%, depending on the length of follow-up and the median age of the patient population.

- Of potent ♂ undergoing 3D-CRT, it was found that the Kaplan Meier potency preservation rates at 1, 2, and 3 years were 100%, 83%, and 63%, respectively.
  [Wilder RB, *Am J Clin Oncol* **23**: 330–333, 2000]
  - 3/7 (43%) of patients who became impotent after 3D-CRT and used sildenafil were subsequently able to achieve erections sufficient for vaginal intercourse.

- In ♂ aged ≤ 65 years who were treated with 3D-CRT the 3- and 6-year potency preservation rates were 73% and 59% vs 85% and 78% in age-matched controls, respectively.
  [Wurzer JC, *Int J Radiat Oncol Biol Phys* **45**: 169, 1999]
  - These rates were similar to previously reported actuarial 1-, 2-, and 3-year rates after 3D-CRT of 92%, 75%, and 66%.
    [Mantz CA, *Int J Radiat Oncol Biol Phys* **37**: 551–557, 1997]

- In ♂ treated with 3D-CRT to a mean dose of 68 Gy who went on to develop erectile dysfunction there was a significant improvement in ability to have an erection, erections firm enough to penetrate, and ability to maintain an erection in patients who received sildenafil (Viagra) vs placebo controls.
  [Inrocci L, *Proc ASTRO* **51**: 139–140, 2001]

- In ♂ who become impotent after EBRT, reported response rates to sildenafil with regard to significant improvement in erectile function range from 66% to 68%.
  [Weber, *Int J Radiat Oncol Biol Phys* **45**: 264–265, 1999]
  [Zelefsky MJ, *Urology* **53**: 775–778, 1999]

- ♂ receiving adjuvant androgen-suppressing therapy with radiation are at greater risk of impotence.
  - Among ♂ potent at baseline, grade 3 impotence ↑ significantly (26.5% vs 20%) with the addition of 6 months of ADT to 70 Gy radiation using 3D-CRT.
    [D'Amico AV, *JAMA* **292**: 821–827, 2004]

- In a study using 3D-CRT to a mean dose of 70.2 Gy, ♂ who were treated with radiation alone were more likely to be potent then were

those who received radiation + ADT, with 1-year potency rates of 56% and 31%, respectively ($p = 0.012$).
[Chen CT, *Int J Radiat Oncol Biol Phys* **50**: 591–595, 2001]

- <u>In conclusion</u>, caution should be exercised when comparing studies of erectile function, because of the differences in terminology, median age of populations studied, and pretreatment function.
  - 3D-CRT demonstrates superior rates of potency preservation over traditional external beam fields.
  - IMRT may prove to surpass 3D-CRT potency-preservation rates; however, long-term follow-up is still needed.
  - ADT, even in the short term, carries a greater risk of impotence.
  - Sildenafil and similar drugs are a reasonable treatment option for ♂ with radiation-induced impotence.

Low dose rate brachytherapy

Urinary toxicity

- Urinary toxicities include ↑ urinary frequency, urgency, retention, dysuria, incontinence, hematuria, and urethral strictures.

- Initial obstructive or irritative urinary symptoms are common after implantation.

- Prolonged symptoms occur in approximately 4% of ♂ with half of them requiring intervention (cystoscopy, TURP, or dilatation).
  [Beyer DC, *Int J Radiat Oncol Biol Phys* **37**: 559–563, 1997]

- In ♂ who underwent iodine-125 seed implantation for low- to intermediate-risk prostate cancer, 46% developed urinary symptoms significant enough at 1 month to require medication.
  [Wallner K, *J Clin Oncol* **14**: 449–453, 1996]
  - These symptoms gradually resolved; at 2 years post-implantation 14% had persistent urinary symptoms graded as Radiation Therapy Oncology Group (RTOG) grade > 2.
  - 8% of ♂ underwent TURP at 2 years.

- Among 145 ♂ who underwent iodine-125 implantation, 3% developed acute urinary retention (grade 3) requiring catheterization.
  [Zelefsky MJ, *J Clin Oncol* **17**: 517–522, 1999]
  - 3% developed acute urinary retention (grade 3) requiring catheterization.
  - No acute grade 4 toxicities were observed.

- 31% had late grade 2 urinary toxicities requiring medication, such as terazosin hydrochloride, that lasted > 1 year, with a median duration of 23 months.

- Late grade 2 urinary toxicities occur in 20–40% of ♂.
  [Zelefsky MJ, *J Clin Oncol* 17: 517–522, 1999]
  [Beyer DC, *Int J Radiat Oncol Biol Phys* 37: 559–563, 1997]
  [Zelefsky MJ, *Int J Radiat Oncol Biol Phys* 47: 1261–1266, 2000]

- The incidence of grade 2 and 3 urinary morbidity is associated with the maximum central urethral dose and with the length of urethra receiving > 400 Gy.
  - In addition, patients with larger prostates have more long-term urinary morbidity.
    [Wallner K, *Int J Radiat Oncol Biol Phys* 32: 465–471, 1995]

- Late urethral strictures occur at a rate of 2–10%.
  [Zelefsky MJ, *J Clin Oncol* 17: 517–522, 1999]
  [Beyer DC, *Int J Radiat Oncol Biol Phys* 37: 559–563, 1997]
  [Zelefsky MJ, *Int J Radiat Oncol Biol Phys* 47: 1261–1266, 2000]

- The median time to development of late urethral strictures is 18 months.
  [Zelefsky MJ, *Int J Radiat Oncol Biol Phys* 47: 1261–1266, 2000]
  [Zelefsky MJ, *J Clin Oncol* 17: 517–522, 1999]

- Of the large series, only one demonstrated any grade 4 late urinary toxicities, at a rate of 0.4%.
  [Zelefsky MJ, *Int J Radiat Oncol Biol Phys* 47: 1261–1266, 2000]

Rectal toxicity

- Rectal toxicities following transperineal seed implantation can include diarrhea, rectal urgency, rectal bleeding, ulceration, or fistula formation.
  - In general, these toxicities occur less frequently than with EBRT.

- 4–12% of ♂ undergoing prostate seed implants develop mild self-limited proctitis, with < 1% developing ulceration and/or fistulas.
  [Howard A, *Brachyther Int* 17: 37–42, 2001]

- In patients undergoing iodine-125 seed implantation for low- to intermediate-risk prostate cancer, an acute rectal toxicity rate of 0% was reported, with 4% developing late grade 2 (rectal bleeding) toxicity, which was treated with conservative measures.
  [Zelefsky MJ, *J Clin Oncol* 17: 517–522, 1999]

- The median duration of late grade 2 symptoms was 8 months and 86% of patients had complete resolution at 36 months.
- No grade 3 or higher toxicities were observed.

- However, another study found that 5/92 ♂ developed radiation-induced rectal ulcers.
  [Wallner K, *J Clin Oncol* **14**: 449–453, 1996]

- Of large series, only one has reported a grade 4 rectal complication (rectourethral fistula), which occurred in 1 ♂.
  [Zelefsky MJ, *Int J Radiat Oncol Biol Phys* **47**: 1261–1266, 2000]

- Rectal function assessment scores after prostate seed implantation correlate with preimplantation bowel movements, tobacco consumption, and median rectal radiation dose.
  [Merrick GS, *Int J Radiation Oncol Biol Phys* **57**: 42–48, 2003]

- Although ♂ implanted with palladium-103 have been shown to have lower rectal doses than those implanted with iodine-125, there is no statistical difference in rectal toxicity rates.

- Rectal bleeding or ulceration is associated with a rectal wall dose > 100 Gy.
  [Wallner K, *Int J Radiat Oncol Biol Phys* **32**: 465–471, 1995]

Erectile dysfunction

- Impotence is a possible complication of transperineal prostate seed implantation.
  - Initial series suggested that brachytherapy may result in superior potency preservation rates over EBRT and RP.

- Earlier reported potency preservation rates after either palladium-103 or iodine-125 → 80–89%.
  [Blasko JC, *Semin Radiat Oncol* **3**: 240–249, 1993]
  [Stock RG, *Int J Radiat Oncol Biol Phys* **35**: 267–272, 1996]
  [Wallner K, *J Clin Oncol* **14**: 449–453, 1996]

- The notion of improved potency rates of brachytherapy over EBRT has recently been challenged.

- 5-year potency rates of 3D-CRT and iodine-125 implantation for low-risk prostate carcinoma were 57% and 47% ($p = 0.52$), respectively.
  [Zelefsky MJ, *J Clin Oncol* **17**: 517–522, 1999]
  - The use of brachytherapy over 3D-CRT did not predict likelihood of impotence.

- The only factors that predicted the development of impotence were 3D-CRT doses > 75.6 Gy and brachytherapy peripheral doses > 160 Gy.

- Potency rates after prostate brachytherapy have been shown to ↓ from 76% when used as monotherapy to 56% when used in combination with EBRT. These rates decrease further when used in combination with ADT.
[Potters L, *Int J Radiat Oncol Biol Phys* **50**: 1235–1242, 2001]

- Prostate brachytherapy-induced impotence is highly correlated with the radiation dose delivered to the bulb of the penis.
[Merrick GS, *Int J Radiat Oncol Biol Phys* **50**: 597–604, 2001]
  - The dose delivered to 50% of the bulb of the penis should be kept < 50 Gy to maximize post-treatment potency.

- The response rate in ♂ with prostate seed-implant-induced impotence to sildenafil is 88%.
[Merrick GS, *Int J Radiat Oncol Biol Phys* **50**: 597–604, 2001]

High dose rate brachytherapy as monotherapy

- High dose rate (HDR) brachytherapy for treatment of prostate cancer has several advantages over low dose rate (LDR) brachytherapy.
  - HDR significantly improves the radiation-dose distribution because of better positional control of the source and the ability to vary the source dwell times, which is done via intraoperative optimization.
  - These advantages offer the opportunity to potentially ↓ treatment-related toxicities.

- Prostate cancer treatment with HDR is still in its infancy, and there is currently a dearth of long-term outcome data.
  - When used as monotherapy, total dose and fraction schemes vary greatly, making interstudy comparisons difficult.

Urinary toxicity

- Common acute toxicities include dysuria, urinary incontinence, urinary retention, urinary urgency or frequency, and hematuria.

- In the five large series where HDR was used as monotherapy, there were no reported grade 3 or higher acute urinary toxicities.
[Yoshioka Y, *Int J Radiat Oncol Biol Phys* **48**: 675–681, 2000]
[Martinez AA, *Int J Radiat Oncol Biol Phys* **49**: 61–69, 2001]

[Vargas C, *J Urol* **174**: 882–887, 2005]
[Grills IA, *J Urol* **171**: 1098–1104, 2004]
[Martin B, *Strahlenther Onkol* **180**: 225–232, 2004]

- Most of lower urinary tract symptoms are temporary, and are managed with alpha-blockers.

- Hematuria, bruising, and pain are rare and easily managed.

- Chronic frequency or dysuria occurs in 2–12% of patients.
  [Morton GC, *Clin Oncol* **17**: 219–227, 2005]

- It has been demonstrated that dysuria and increased urinary frequency or urgency occur statistically more frequently in those patients undergoing LDR prostate implantation vs HDR implantation.
  [Grills IA, *J Urol* **171**: 1098–1104, 2004]

- The most commonly reported late side-effect is urethral stricture, which occurs at a rate of 0–14%.
  [Pellizzon AC, *J Urol* **171**: 1105–1108, 2004]

- Urethral strictures most commonly occur in the bulbar urethra, and are associated with use of midline needles, previous TURP, and older age.

- The overall risk of incontinence is 1%, and occurs almost exclusively in patients who have undergone TURP.
  [Galalae RM, *Int J Radiat Oncol Biol Phys* **58**: 1048–1055, 2004]

- Risk factors for ≥ grade 2 urinary toxicity (statistically significant).
  [Vargas C, *J Urol* **174**: 882–887, 2005]
  - Use of ≥ 14 needles.
  - Prostate volume > 38 cm^3.
  - Neoadjuvant hormone therapy.

Rectal toxicity

- Acute toxicities include diarrhea, rectal pain, and rectal bleeding.

- Acute rectal toxicities are rare, and usually occur in those patients who have received accompanying EBRT.

- In all large series there have been no reported grade 3 or higher acute gastrointestinal toxicities.
  - Grade 1 or 2 acute gastrointestinal toxicities occur in 19% of patients.
    [Yoshioka Y, *Int J Radiat Oncol Biol Phys* **48**: 675–681, 2000]

- Long-term rectal toxicities are rare, occurring at a rate of 0–4%, and include diarrhea, proctitis, and bleeding.

- The 3-year, grade 2 rectal toxicity rate has been shown to be 1%, with no grade 3 or higher toxicities reported.
  [Vargas C, J Urol **174**: 882–887, 2005]
  [Yoshioka Y, Int J Radiat Oncol Biol Phys **48**: 675–681, 2000]

- Late rectal ulceration and rectourethral fistula are rare, occurring in 0–1.7% of patients.

- Late rectal toxicities have been demonstrated to be similar with HDR and LDR implants.
  [Vargas C, J Urol **174**: 882–887, 2005]
  [Grills IA, J Urol **171**: 1098–1104, 2004]

- Rectal pain has been shown to occur more frequently with LDR implants (20%) than with HDR implants (6%).
  [Grills IA, J Urol **171**: 1098–1104, 2004]

Erectile dysfunction

- Impotence has been shown to occur at a rate of 16–18%.

- Two series comparing impotency between HDR and LDR monotherapies demonstrated an approximately 70% decrease in the impotency rate with the use of HDR over LDR.
  [Grills IA, J Urol **171**: 1098–1104, 2004]
  [Vargas C, J Urol **174**: 882–887, 2005]
  - This difference was statistically significant in one series ($p = 0.002$) but not in the other ($p = 0.062$).

Cryotherapy

- There has been a documented increased toxicity with cryotherapy, especially when used as salvage after radiation therapy.

- Recent improvements in technique, including urethral warming during the procedure, have reduced the complication rate.

- There has been little long-term follow-up, and whether newer approaches will reduce late complications is unclear.

Urinary toxicity

- Urinary side-effects include incontinence, hematuria, urinary tract infection, obstructive uropathy, and rectourethral fistulas.

- In general, after the procedure patients are discharged with either a suprapubic or urethral catheter, which remains in place for 2 weeks.

- The rate of urinary incontinence has been reported to be 70–95%.
  [De La Taille A, *BJU Int* **85**: 281–286, 2000]
  [Pisters L, *J Urol* **157**: 921–925, 1997]

- Urinary incontinence occurs more frequently in salvage patients than those treated primarily with cryotherapy.
  [Anastasis AG, *J Cancer Res Clin Oncol* **129**: 676–682, 2003]

- The use of an effective urethral warming catheter is associated with a decrease in urinary incontinence.
  [Perotte P, *J Urol* **162**: 398–402, 1999]
  - The rate of urinary incontinence improves with time, and can resolve in 47% of cases with the use of urethral warming.
    [Perotte P, *J Urol* **162**: 398–402, 1999]

- Other urinary toxicities include hematuria (6%) and urinary infections (3%).
  [De La Taille A, *BJU Int* **85**: 281–286, 2000]

- Urinary obstructive symptoms occur in approximately 65% of patients.
  [Pisters L, *J Urol* **157**: 921–925, 1997]

- A serious potential complication of cryotherapy is the formation of a rectourethral fistula. These fistulas occur in 0–11% of patients.
  [Chin J, *J Urol* **165**: 1937–1941, 2001]
  [Pisters L, *J Urol* **157**: 921–925, 1997]
  [Bales GT, *Urology* **46**: 676–680, 1995]

- Before the introduction of urethral warming devices, tissue sloughing was a problem.
  [Bales GT, *Urology* **46**: 676–680, 1995]

Erectile dysfunction

- Impotence is a significant problem post-cryotherapy, and occurs in 72–100% of patients.
  [Anastasis AG, *J Cancer Res Clin Oncol* **129**: 676–682, 2003]
  [Pisters L, *J Urol* **157**: 921–925, 1997]

- The predicted probability of maintaining erectile function after cryotherapy is only 0.13, compared with after brachytherapy (0.76), brachytherapy + EBRT (0.60), EBRT (0.60), nerve-sparing RP (0.34), and RP (0.25).
  [Robinson JW, *Int J Radiat Oncol Biol Phys* **54**: 1063–1068, 2002]

- The impotence rate is higher when cryotherapy is used as a salvage therapy as opposed to a primary therapy.

- Impotence has been shown to increase significantly from 77% to 92% with the use of two freeze–thaw cycles as opposed to one.
  [Perotte P, J Urol 162: 398–402, 1999]

Chronic pelvic, rectal or perineal pain

- Pelvic, rectal, and perineal pain is a frequent complication that occurs in 8–44% of patients, and in one series it interfered with normal activity in 38% of patients.
  [Cespedes RD, J Urol 157: 237–240, 1997]
  [Perotte P, J Urol 162: 398–402, 1999]
  [Pisters L, J Urol 157: 921–925, 1997]

- Patients treated without a urethral warming catheter have a statistically significant higher rate of pain (70% vs 34%).
  [Perotte P, J Urol 162: 398–402, 1999]

Androgen-suppression therapy

[Holzbeierlein, J Curr Opin Urol 14: 177–183, 2004]

- Initially, androgen deprivation was accomplished by orchiectomy; this was then replaced by estrogens.
  - For reasons of poor patient acceptance, as well as thromboembolic and cardiovascular events, estrogens were later mostly abandoned and supplanted by luteinizing hormone releasing hormone (LHRH) agonists.

Hot flashes

- Usually described as intense warmth of the upper body and face lasting for a few minutes, but can last for hours.

- Hot flashes are one of the most common side-effects associated with ADT and can occur in up to 80% of patients using LHRH agonists.
  [Karling P, J Urol 152: 1170–1173, 1994]
  [Charig CR, Urology 33: 175–178, 1989]
  - Although spontaneous resolution of hot flashes can occur, many patients will suffer from them for as long as they are on ADT.

- Triggers include change in position, heat, stress, and ingestion of hot liquids.
  [Smith JA, Oncology 10: 1319–1322, 1996]

- Transdermal estrogen results in improvement in 83% of patients.
  [Gerber GS, *Urology* **55**: 97–101, 2000]
  [Miller JI, *Urology* **40**: 499–502, 1992]
  - Oral diethylstilbesterol has a reported complete response rate and partial response rate of 70% and 20%, respectively.

- Medroxyprogesterone acetate and megestrol acetate are both progestins with a reported efficacy of 80–85%.
  [Loprinzi CL, *N Engl J Med* **331**: 347–352, 1994]

- Clonidine was initially thought to be useful in the treatment of hot flashes, but randomized studies demonstrated no advantage over placebo.
  [Loprinzi CL, *J Urol* **151**: 634–636, 1994]

- Selective serotonin reuptake inhibitors reportedly decrease symptoms of hot flashes.
  - Venlafaxine, in particular, has shown some promise, but has yet to be tested in placebo-controlled trials.

Osteoporosis

- Osteoporosis and ↓ bone mineral density have been demonstrated in ♂ undergoing orchiectomy or taking LHRH agonists.
  [Stoch SA, *J Clin Endocrinol Metab* **86**: 27–37, 2001]

- The 5- and 10-year risks for osteoporotic hip fractures in ♂ on LHRH agonists are 5% and 20%, respectively.
  [Morote J, *Eur Urol* **44**: 661–665, 2003]

- In ♂ on LHRH agonists who are > 75 years old there is a 30% associated mortality with hip fractures.
  [Townsend MF, *Cancer* **79**: 545–550, 1997]

- Preventive measures include resistance exercise, and calcium and vitamin D supplementation.

- Current recommended doses of calcium and vitamin D are 1,200 mg/day and 400 IU/day, respectively.

- Bisphosphonates are an option for both the prevention and the treatment of ADT osteoporosis.
  - Alendronate has been shown to increase bone mineral density in ♂ with osteoporosis.
  - Zolendronate has been shown to increase bone mineral density and reduce skeletal-related events in ♂ on ADT.

[Saad F, *J Natl Cancer Inst* **94**: 1458–1468, 2002]
[Smith MR, *J Urol* **169**: 2008–2012, 2003]

Anemia

- Testosterone and dihydrotestosterone are important stimulants for erythropoietin production and erythroid precursors.

- ADT anemia is usually normocytic, normochromic anemia.

- ~ 90% of patients on complete androgen deprivation experience a ≥ 10% drop in their hemoglobin.
  - Drops in hemoglobin can occur in a month from initiation of ADT and reach a nadir at 5.6 months.
  - Resolution after discontinuation of ADT frequently takes > 1 year.
    [Strum SB, *Br J Urol* **79**: 993–941, 1997]

- There have been no clinical trials evaluating erythropoietin replacement therapy in the treatment of ADT anemia, but it has been used off label.

Sexual dysfunction

- Sexual dysfunction occurs in most ♂ on ADT.

- In ♂ taking LHRH agonists, decreased libido usually occurs within the first year.

- Finasteride and flutamide have been used in combination as ADT for advanced prostate cancer.
  - While these drugs demonstrated initial preservation of potency, with longer follow-up there was a reduction in potency and libido. Further evaluation of this therapy is needed.
    [Brufsky A, *Urology* **49**: 913–920, 1997]

Cognitive function

- Hypogonadal elderly ♂ without prostate cancer have been shown to have ↓ cognition.
  - This patient population has been shown to have improved spatial ability, verbal memory, and fluency with testosterone replacement.
    [Tan RS, *J Androl* **23**: 45–46, 2002]

- ↓ in memory, attention, and executive function have been demonstrated after 6 months of ADT.
  [Green HJ, 23: 45–46, 2002]

- – Another study comparing ♂ on 12 months of ADT with healthy controls showed no difference in cognitive deficits between the two groups.
  [Salimen E, *Br J Cancer* **89**: 971–976, 2003]

- Although it is reasonable to conclude that long-term ADT causes impaired cognitive function, there is still dispute regarding the effects of short-term ADT.

Body composition changes

[Williams MB, *J Urol* **173**: 1067–1071, 2005]

- Weight gain is a common side-effect with ADT.

- Patients on combined androgen blockade have a mean weight gain of 6 kg.
  [Higano CS, *Urology* **48**: 800–804, 1996]
  - – Weight and body mass index ↑ by 2.4% after 48 weeks.
    [Smith MR, *J Clin Endocrinol Metab* **87**: 599–602, 2002]

- The etiology of ADT weight gain is related to decreased activity secondary to fatigue, changes in appetite, and a decrease in muscle mass.

- ↓ in lean muscle mass and increases in body fat are believed to be directly correlated with a drop in serum testosterone.

- Although there is no documented correlation between current day ADT and cardiovascular events, total cholesterol and triglycerides have been shown to increase by 9% and 26.5%, respectively, in ♂ on ADT.

Chemotherapy

[Beer TM, *Semin Urol Oncol* **19**: 222–230, 2001]
[Beer TM, *Urol Clin North Am* **31**: 331–352, 2004]

- Chemotherapy has gained popularity only recently in the treatment of prostate cancer, and therefore the prevention and treatment of chemotherapy-related toxicities have not yet been well studied.

- Mechanisms of chemotherapy are not cancer specific. Normal tissues, especially those undergoing rapid proliferation, are vulnerable to these cytotoxic drugs.

- Toxicities of single agents, and both agents when used in combination, must be taken into account.
  - – These effects may be additive; however, this is not always the case.

- There may be patient-specific factors that effect chemotherapy-related toxicities.
  - These may include age, extent of cancer, other comorbidities, or prior chemotherapy/radiation therapy/radiopharmaceuticals, or other myelosuppressive medications, which may all be associated with diminished bone marrow reserves.
  [Mauch P, Int J Radiat Oncol Biol Phys 31: 1319–1339, 1995]

Doxorubicin + estramustine

[Culine S, Am J Clin Oncol 21: 470–474, 1998]

- Almost all patients developed either grade 2 or 3 alopecia.

- 38% of patients developed grade 3 or 4 neutropenia.

- 25% of patients developed grade 2 stomatitis.

- There was no documented heart toxicity.

Mitoxantrone + prednisone

[Tannock IF, J Clin Oncol 14: 1756–1764, 1996]

- Approved for use in androgen-independent prostate cancer.

- 30% of patients have some nausea, with severe nausea and vomiting occurring infrequently.

- 76% of patients had no hair loss, with the remaining having partial loss.

- ~ 50% of patients have neutropenia (< 1,000 neutrophils/mm^3).
  - In one study the incidence of neutropenic fever was 1.1%.
  [Berry W, J Urol 168: 2439–2443, 2002]

- ≥ Grade 3 gastrointestinal complications occur in 5% of patients, compared with 2% of patients taking prednisone only.

- Cardiac toxicity, including congestive heart failure, is a rare but severe complication that is associated with higher cumulative doses of mitoxantrone.

Etoposide + estramustine

[Pienta KJ, J Clin Oncol 12: 2005–2012, 1994]

- In Phase II studies the most common side-effects included fatigue, nipple tenderness, nausea, and fluid overload (edema).

- Initial studies demonstrated an incidence of grade 3 or 4 hematologic toxicity of 24%, with a similar incidence of thrombocytopenia.
  - More recent data have shown infrequent hematologic toxicity, with no episodes of neutropenic fever.
  - This discrepancy may be, in part, due to a lower estramustine dose. [Vaishampayan U, *Am J Clin Oncol* **27**: 550–554, 2004]
- Nearly all patients experience alopecia.

5-Fluorouracil and leucovorin (Eastern Cooperative Oncology Group (ECOG) E1889)

[Berlin J, *Am J Clin Oncol* **21**: 171–176, 1998]

- 60% of patients experienced at least one grade 3 or 4 toxicity.
- The most common side-effects were gastroenterologic and hematologic.
- Grade 3 and 4 nausea, vomiting, diarrhea, and stomatitis were frequent.
- 36% of patients experienced grade 3 or 4 leukopenia or anemia.
- 8% of patients developed some form of thrombophlebitis.

Docetaxel monotherapy

- When given on a 21-day basis docetaxel monotherapy is associated with frequent neutropenia.
  [Picus J, *Semin Oncol* **26**: 14–18, 1999]
  [Beer TC, *Ann Oncol* **26**: 1273–1279, 2001]
  - Hematologic toxicity is less with weekly administration.
- Protracted treatment with weekly docetaxel result in frequent nail toxicity.

Docetaxel + estramustine

[Savarese DM, *J Clin Oncol* **19**: 2509–2516, 2001]

- Myelosuppression, gastrointestinal toxicity, and thromboembolic events are a concern with these regimens.
- Hematologic toxicity is frequent, and ~ 50% of patients experience grade 3 or 4 neutropenia.
- 20% of patients developed neuropathy.

- Nausea, vomiting, and diarrhea occurred in 18%, 13%, and 25% of patients, respectively.

- Thromboembolic complications occur in 6–10% of patients; however, another study using a lower dose of estramustine in combination with warfarin reported no such complications.
  [Sinibaldi VJ, *Cancer* **94**: 1457–1465, 2002]
  [Copur MS, *Semin Oncol* **28**: 16–21, 2001]

- When suramin was added to this regimen, hematologic and gastro-intestinal toxicities remained the same; however, 14% of patients developed rash.
  [Safarinejad MR, *Urol Oncol* **23**: 93–101, 2005]

Paclitaxel + estramustine

[Hudes GR, *J Clin Oncol* **15**: 3156–3163, 1997]

- Common side-effects include nausea, gynecomastia, and edema.

- 79% of patients developed nausea, 52% edema, and 39% gynecomastia.

- ≥ Grade 3 leukopenia in 21% of patients.

- 9% of patients developed thrombosis.

Paclitaxel + epirubicin

[Neri B, *Anticancer Drugs* **16**: 63–66, 2005]

- Common side-effects include fatigue, nausea/vomiting, hematologic effects, and alopecia.

- The only reported grade 3 or higher toxicities were anemia and leuko-penia, with 6% of each. There were no incidences of neutropenic fever.

Treatment of chemotherapy-related side-effects.

Nausea and vomiting

- Patient-related risk factors that increase the risk for chemotherapy-related nausea and vomiting include minimal alcohol use, age < 50 years, nausea with previous chemotherapy, and a history of motion sickness.
  [Therapeutic ASHP, *Am J Health Syst Pharm* **56**: 729–764, 1999]

- Most regimens used for prostate cancer are not strong emetogenics.

- First-line agents in the treatment and prevention of nausea and vomiting include corticosteroids, dopamine inhibitors, and serotonin inhibitors.

Mucositis

- Many chemotherapies cause breakdown of the oral mucosa.

- Maintaining good oral hygiene, using a soft toothbrush and mild toothpaste, minimal flossing, minimizing tobacco and alcohol use, and regular saline or baking soda rinses, is strongly encouraged.

- Initial symptomatic management includes topical medications such as benzocaine, lidocaine, phenol, Magic Mouthwash (lidocaine, diphenhydramine (Benadryl), nystatin, tetracycline, and hydrocortisone) or triple mix (Benadryl, Maalox, and lidocaine (Xylocaine)).

- In most cases systemic pain medication is required, initially with non-steroidal anti-inflammatory drugs, and progressing to long-acting narcotics with short-acting agents for breakthrough pain.

- Sucralfate (Carafate) slurry may augment the healing process.

- Superinfection with *Candida* can be treated with fluconazole, ketoconazole, or nystatin suspension.
    - When fungal infections occur in the background of mucositis, protracted treatment courses are required.

Anemia and neutropenia

- Anemia and associated fatigue are common side-effects to both ADT and antineoplastic agents used in prostate cancer.

- The use of growth factors eliminates the need for transfusion and ↓ fatigue.

- In prostate cancer the two most commonly used growth factors are epoetin-α and darbepoetin-α.

- Darbepoetin is generally given every 2 weeks, whereas epoetin is given on a weekly basis.

- The use of growth factors for neutropenia is to prevent neutropenic fevers or avoid dose ↓.
    - Sargramostim, filgrastim, and pegfilgrastim are commonly used agents.

26

Follow-up of patients after treatment of localized prostate cancer

Recurrence after primary therapy

- Although radical prostatectomy and radiation therapy for localized prostate cancer are sometimes referred to as 'definitive therapy', a significant number of patients will have cancer recurrence after surgery.

- Radiation therapy may consist of:
  - External beam radiation therapy.
  - Intraprostatic radiation seeds.
  - A combination of both.

- Overall recurrence rates after radiation therapy are similar to those after prostatectomy.

- 40% will recur overall.
  [Hull GW, J Urol 167: 528–534, 2002]
  - 20–25% of patients will have a prostate-specific antigen (PSA) recurrence at 5 years post-treatment.
    [Catalona WJ, J Urol 152(5 Pt 2): 1837–1842, 1994]
  - 5–27% of patients will recur > 5 years after treatment.
    [Pound CR, JAMA 281(17): 1591–1597, 1999]
    [Ward JF, J Urol 170(5): 1872–1876, 2003]

- PSA recurrence tends to precede clinical cancer recurrence by about 6–8 years.
  [Sofer M, J Urol 167(6): 2453–2456, 2002]

- One-third of patients with PSA recurrence will develop clinical recurrence.

- Most recurrences occur within 5 years of prostatectomy.

- This chapter centers on the follow-up of patients following treatment for localized prostate cancer, as well as the treatment options available after recurrence.

Follow-up protocol following primary therapy

- Although follow-up schedules differ, many clinicians recommend the following:
  - Every 3 months for 1–2 years, then
  - Every 6 months for 3–4 years, then
  - Annually.

- Patients should be followed regularly with a PSA measurement performed at, or prior to, the office visit.

- PSA should remain at undetectable levels after prostatectomy, as very little PSA is produced outside the prostate.

- After radiation therapy, PSA usually does not $\downarrow$ to undetectable levels, but should reach a nadir and then stabilize.
  - The PSA typically $\downarrow$ usually for 12–18 months following treatment.
  - The PSA may continue to $\downarrow$ for up to 5 years.
  - The likelihood of recurrence may be predicted by the PSA nadir:
    - Nadir < 0.5 is desirable, with an 80–90% recurrence-free rate.
    - Nadir > 1 suggests a lower recurrence-free rate of 0–40%.

- A digital rectal examination (DRE) is not necessary after prostatectomy, but is often used following radiation therapy.
  [Pound CR, JAMA **281**(17): 1591–1597, 1999]
  - The prostate should feel flat and fixed after radiation treatment.

- Imaging studies are also not necessary in patients with an undetectable PSA.

Biochemical recurrence

- PSA-only recurrence, called biochemical recurrence, usually precedes clinical recurrence by 6–8 years.

- A PSA recurrence does not, in itself, indicate whether the recurrence is local or systemic (see the following section).

- The PSA cut-off to be used for defining recurrence after prostatectomy is a subject of some mild controversy.

[Freedland SJ, *Urology* **61**(2): 365–369, 2003]
- A PSA of 0.2 ng/ml is used by most clinicians as a cut-off point.
- Many feel 0.4 ng/ml PSA is more appropriate, for the following two reasons:
  - Most patients with a PSA of 0.4 ng/ml do not have a continued PSA ↑.
  - Residual benign prostatic hyperplasia BPH tissue left behind at the time of surgery may result in a slight amount of PSA production over time. This does not represent cancer recurrence.

- PSA recurrence after radiation therapy was defined by the American Society of Therapeutic Radiology and Oncology (ASTRO) criteria: [Cox JD, American Society for Therapeutic Radiology and Oncology Consensus Panel, *J Clin Oncol* **17**(4): 1155–1163 (review), 1999]
  - Three consecutive ↑ in PSA over the nadir.
  - PSA measurements should be made 6 months apart.
  - After a patient is deemed as having a recurrence, the date of recurrence is backdated to the midpoint between the PSA nadir and the first PSA ↑.

- The more recent RTOG-ASTRO Phoenix Consensus Conference definition has replaced the previous ASTRO definition, and correlates better with future risk of clinical progression. The definition of PSA recurrence after radiation is an increase of 2 ng/ml or more above the nadir.
[Roach M, *Int J Radiat Oncol Biol Phys* **65**(4): 965–974, 2006]

- PSA bounce often occurs in patients who have had radiotherapy.
  - This is a transient ↑ in the PSA after radiation therapy.
  - Occurs more often following brachytherapy.
  - Seen in ~ 17–30% of patients, at an average of 19.4 months post-treatment.
  - More common in younger men, men with a higher implant dose, and men with larger prostates.
  [Stock RG, *Int J Radiat Oncol Biol Phys* **56**(2): 448–453, 2003]
  - PSA bounce does not represent recurrence.

Predictors of recurrence

- The chances of a patient developing a recurrence depend on the pathologic stage.
- Pathologic factors that ↑ the likelihood of recurrence include:
  - Extracapsular extension.

- Seminal vesicle invasion (50–70% recurrence rate).
- (+) lymph nodes (LNs).
- Tumor volume > 20%.
- (+) margins.
  [Sofer M, J Urol **167**(6): 2453–2456, 2002]
  - 1 margin → 25% recurrence rate.
  - 2 margins → 30% recurrence rate.
  - The location of the (+) margin is <u>not</u> important.

- When counseling patients, clinicians often use the Partin tables, which attempt to predict pathologic findings based on the Gleason score, clinical stage, and pretreatment PSA.
  [Partin AW, JAMA **277**: 1445–1451, 1999]

- After surgery, the pathology results can help guide patient counseling regarding the probability of recurrence.

- After radiation therapy, only clinical factors can be used to discuss the probability of recurrence.

- Many clinicians divide patients with clinically localized cancer into three groups, with various risks of recurrence following treatment.
  [D'Amico AV, J Clin Oncol **21**(11): 2163–2172, 2003]
  - Low risk (15% 5-year PSA recurrence rate).
    - Clinical stage T_{1c}–T_{2a}.
    - Gleason score ≤ 6.
    - PSA ≤ 10 ng/ml.
  - Intermediate risk (50% 5-year PSA recurrence rate).
    - Clinical stage T_{2b}.
    - PSA 10–20 ng/ml.
    - Gleason score 7.
  - High risk (66% 5-year PSA recurrence rate).
    - Clinical stage T_{2c}.
    - PSA > 20 ng/ml.
    - Gleason score ≥ 8.

- Race and age do not appear to be predictors of recurrence.
  [Tewari A, BJU Int **96**(1): 29–33, 2005]
  [Gomez P, Cancer **100**(8): 1628–1632, 2004]

Distinguishing local from systemic recurrence

- Once a patient has been diagnosed as having a recurrence following treatment, the clinician must determine whether the recurrence is local or systemic.

- The distinction is important because patients with local recurrence only are candidates for salvage procedures.
  - Salvage prostatectomy after radiation treatment.
  - Salvage radiotherapy after prostatectomy.

- In the absence of clinical metastases, the urologist must use clinical judgment, after reviewing the patient's pathology results and PSA parameters, to define the recurrence as local or systemic.

- PSA dynamics may be an indication of local vs systemic disease.
  - Timing of the PSA rise.
  - The length of time necessary for the PSA to double (PSA doubling time (PSADT)).
    [Patel A, J Urol **158**(4): 1441–1445, 1997]
    - < 6 months is indicative of systemic metastasis.
    - > 10 months → 76% chance of remaining disease free.
    - < 10 months → 35% chance of remaining disease free.
      [Pound CR, JAMA **281**(17): 1591–1597, 1999]
  - A Gleason score of 8–10 is more likely to recur systemically.

- If the PSA level is undetectable no DRE is necessary; however, a rise in PSA may provoke a rectal examination.

- If a nodule is detected in the prostatic fossa, this may be biopsied.
  - The sensitivity and specificity of a DRE in detecting biopsy-proven local recurrence are 72.4% and 64.8%.
    [Naya Y, Urology **66**(2): 350–355, 2005]

- After radiation therapy, the prostate can also be biopsied to look for viable tumor.
  - Biopsy should be performed at least 18 months after radiotherapy.
    - Radiotherapy may take up to 18 months for complete regression of cancer.

- ProstaScint is a nuclear medicine study that uses radiolabeled tracers to try to identify whether recurrence exists locally in the prostate or prostatic fossa, or whether there is spread to the LNs or bones.
  [Kahn D, ProstaScint Study Group, J Urol **159**(6): 2041–2046; 2046–2047 (discussion), 1998]
  - It has limited use at present as it is insufficiently sensitive and specific.

- Imaging studies have not been helpful.
  [Okotie OT, J Urol **171**(6 Pt 1): 2260–2264, 2004]

- Bone scans are unlikely to be (+), and are not recommended, for people with a PSA < 7 ng/ml after recurrence.
  [Gomez P, BJU Int **94**(3): 299–302, 2004]

Treatment following recurrence

Local disease

After prostatectomy

- Treatment of localized disease following prostatectomy is salvage radiotherapy.

- Risks of salvage radiotherapy include:
  - Increasing likelihood of impotence.
  - Possibly worsening voiding symptoms.
  - Further devascularizing tissue, leading to complications.
  - Possible hemorrhagic cystitis.

- Benefits are that some patients can be cured.
  [Kattan MW, *J Clin Oncol* **21**(24): 4568–4571, 2003]
  - Patients with no adverse features have had a 4-year progression-free survival rate of 77%.
    [Stephenson AJ, JAMA **291**(11): 1325–1332, 2004]

- Patients who are more likely to progress after salvage radiotherapy have:
  - Gleason score 8–10 (hazard ratio (HR) 2.6).
  - Pre-radiation PSA > 2.0 ng/ml (HR 2.3).
  - (–) surgical margins (HR 1.9).
  - PSADT < 10 months (HR 1.7).
  - Seminal vesicle invasion (HR 1.4).

- The ASTRO consensus panel suggests that the highest efficacy of salvage radiotherapy occurs when given at the lowest PSA level.
  - A PSA of 1.5 ng/ml is suggested to be the highest value where efficacy is seen.
    [Cox JD, American Society for Therapeutic Radiology and Oncology Consensus Panel, *J Clin Oncol* **17**(4): 1155–1163 (review), 1999]

- Some experts strongly suggest that patients with (+) margins after surgery be considered for salvage radiotherapy, even in the face of high Gleason grade disease and low PSADT.
  - Rates of 4-year disease-free survival as high as 80% have been shown in this cohort of patients.
    [Stephenson AJ, JAMA **291**(11): 1325–1332, 2004]

After radiotherapy

- Following radiotherapy, salvage prostatectomy may be a viable option.

- Risks of salvage prostatectomy are:
  [Ward JF, *J Urol* **173**(4): 1156–1160, 2005]
  - High risk of rectal injury: 2–15%.
  - High chance of bladder neck contracture: 22–30%.
  - Higher rate of incontinence: 50–60%.
  - Higher risk of impotence: 28% potency rates in the best hands.
  - Difficult surgery, often involving higher blood loss.

- Long-term outcomes following salvage prostatectomy.
  [Bianco FJ Jr, *Int J Radiat Oncol Biol Phys* **62**(2): 448–453, 2005]
  - Overall 5-year progression-free survival → 55%.
  - Median time to progression after surgery → 6.4 years.

- Patients who stand to benefit are:
  [Bianco FJ Jr, *Int J Radiat Oncol Biol Phys* **62**(2): 448–453, 2005]
  - Younger patients.
  - Presurgery PSA < 10 ng/ml.
    - For PSA < 4.0 ng/ml → 86% progression-free survival.
    - For PSA 4–10 ng/ml → 55% progression-free survival.
      For PSA > 10 ng/ml → 37% progression-free survival.

- Salvage cryotherapy and salvage brachytherapy have also been studied in patients with recurrence.
  - Salvage cryotherapy.
    - 75% 1-year progression-free rate.
    - 40% biochemical-disease-free rate over 5-years.
      [Chin JL, *Technol Cancer Res Treat* **4**(2): 211–216, 2005]
    - Complications:
      [Han KR, *J Urol* **170**(4 Pt 1): 1126–1130, 2003]
      - Impotence: 87%.
      - Tissue sloughing: 5%.
      - Incontinence: 3%.
      - Urinary retention: 3%.
  - Salvage brachytherapy: there is currently a paucity of data on this therapy.

Systemic recurrence

- The mainstay of treatment for systemic recurrence of prostate cancer is androgen-deprivation therapy.

- Androgen-deprivation therapy can consist of several options.
  - Surgical castration.
  - Luteinizing hormone releasing hormone (LHRH) agonist use.

- – LHRH antagonist use.
- – Antiandrogen use.
- – Combined, or maximum, androgen blockade.
- – Estrogens.

- Surgical castration provides the best option for non-compliant patients, eliminating the testicular source of androgens.

- LHRH agonist therapy is essentially medical castration. By providing a constant source of LHRH (rather than the physiologic pulsatile release of LHRH), the body ceases production of luteinizing hormone (LH).
  - SIDE-EFFECTS OF LHRH AGONISTS:
    - – Lethargy, fatigue.
    - – Hot flashes.
    - – ↓ libido.
    - – Loss of lean muscle tissue.
    - – ↑ body fat.
    - – Anemia.
    - – ↓ bone density.

- Antiandrogens block the action of androgens on their receptors as opposed to blocking the actual production of androgens.
  - Can be used in conjunction with LHRH agonists, but have been used as monotherapy at higher doses.
    [Iversen, P, J Urol 170(6 Pt 2): S48–S52 (review), discussion S52–S54 (discussion), 2003]
    - – Similar survival benefit.
    - – Higher cost.
    - – Better for younger men who desire to keep their libido.
  - SIDE-EFFECTS:
    - – Breast pain.
    - – Gynecomastia.
    - – Diarrhea/gastrointestinal upset.
    - – Liver inflammation.

- Combined androgen blockade is the combination of an LHRH agonist with an antiandrogen.
  - – Not all androgen production is under the control of LH.
  - – Antiandrogens block the 10–15% of androgens produced by the adrenal gland.
  - – Meta-analysis has shown a 2.5–3% survival benefit of using combined therapy.
  - – ↑ the cost of treatment and the risk of side-effects.

Timing of therapy

- There is considerable debate over when to start androgen deprivation after systemic recurrence.
  - Some suggest beginning treatment after biochemical recurrence.
  - Others promote waiting until the development of clinical metastasis.

- No prospective study has proven a survival benefit to early androgen deprivation, except in the following situations:
  - (+) LNs at prostatectomy → 25% survival benefit.
    [Messing EM, N Engl J Med 341(24): 1781–1788, 1999]
  - In conjunction with radiotherapy for locally advanced disease.
    [Bolla M, Lancet 360(9327): 103–106, 2002]

- Early androgen-deprivation therapy has been shown to prolong time to onset of metastasis and symptoms secondary to prostate cancer.

- Evidence is mounting that early treatment with hormone-deprivation therapy may improve survival in patients with locally advanced prostate cancer.
  [Moul JW, J Urol 171(3): 1141–1147, 2004]

Metastatic disease

- Patients most at risk of developing distant metastases have:
  - High-grade disease (Gleason score 8–10).
  - Rapid PSADT (< 6 months).
  - Early recurrence after treatment.

- Treatment with androgen-deprivation agents is first-line treatment in newly diagnosed patients.

- Patients developing metastasis after development of hormone-resistant disease should still be maintained on hormone therapy.

- Focus on the prevention of symptoms secondary to progressive local disease:
  - Urinary retention/difficulty urinating.
  - Ureteral obstruction.
  - Rectal obstruction.

- Systemic metastases may result in:
  - ↑ pain from bone metastases.
  - Cauda equina syndrome.
    - Urologic emergency.

- The PSA level is of limited value in patients with metastatic disease; however, it may act as a surrogate marker to show the effectiveness of treatment agents.

- Chemotherapy agents are available, and have recently been shown to improve survival.
  - Combination of docetaxel and estramustine with steroids.
    [Petrylak DP, N Engl J Med **351**(15): 1513–1520, 2004]
    [Tannock IF, N Engl J Med **351**(15): 1502–1512, 2004]
  - Patients given q 3 weekly docetaxel had an HR for death of 0.76–0.80.

- Samarium and strontium treatments have a palliative benefit in many patients.
  [Serafini AN, J Clin Oncol **16**(4): 1574–1581, 1998]
  - 62–72% of patients had a palliative benefit from samarium treatment.
  - 30% of patients had complete relief of pain by 4 weeks.
  - Bone marrow suppression is a side-effect, but is mild and reversible.

Index